RIGHT TOOL FOR THE JOB

RIGHT TOOL FOR THE JOB

A Memoir of Manly Concerns

MARK GOLDBLATT

LIBERTY ISLAND

978-1-5040-4224-6

Liberty Island Media Group
New York, NY
www.LibertyIslandMag.com

Distributed in 2016 by Open Road Distribution
180 Maiden Lane
New York, NY 10038
www.openroadmedia.com

FOR INGER STEVENS,

the shikse's shikse,

R.I.P.

CONTENTS

PREFACE

The book you're holding in your hand is, as Huck Finn once said, "mostly a true book, with some stretchers." I'm supposing you *are* holding the book in your hand, either in paper-and-ink form, or encoded in binaries and magicked into an electronic device, but even in the unlikely event you're ingesting this a hundred years from now as a lozenge, you're still going to find a few things that are hard to swallow. But they did happen. With stretchers.

Huck Finn of course is a famous fictional character. Whereas the Mark Goldblatt who inhabits these pages is a creature of flesh and blood, not famous but not altogether obscure, subject to the usual set of human frailties whereby recollection is clouded by time and warped by ego. I have tried, insofar as possible, not to misremember to my advantage. When the seltzer goes down anyone's pants, I want it to be mine. Nonetheless, there is more than enough here to give offense. Therefore: To friends, relatives, and occasional lovers who find themselves, or facsimiles of themselves, in the narratives that follow, I apologize abjectly and in advance.

Do I flatter myself to think a few readers may know me already . . . as a novelist, or a children's book author, or a right-of-center political columnist, or (that rarest of rarities) a tenured conservative at a public university? If fame can be gauged by Google searches, I seem to rank somewhere between a middling rapper and an Investigation Discovery murder-porn victim. It's enough. Several years ago, I was riding the subway in Manhattan when I noticed that the woman sitting across from me was reading one of my novels. Yeah, I was feeling pretty good about myself right then, debating whether or not to ask if she wanted an autograph. Before I could decide, however, she got off . . . and the British actor Jeremy Irons got on and took her seat. Every atom of his being, the look on his face, the angle of his head, the slouch of his shoulders, the fold of his arms, the tightness of his jacket, seemed to cry out, "Please, please, *please*, for once, let me ride the train in peace!" Real celebrity carries a cost. And he was only Jeremy Irons. Not Sean P. Puff Diddy Daddy Combs . . .

So, for the record, I'm neither Sean P. Puff Diddy Daddy Combs nor Jeremy Irons. I ride the train safely cocooned in anonymity, content with my lot. Why wouldn't I be? I was born a grand-prize winner in that greatest of all secular lotteries—I'm an American—and have arrived at late middle age in decent health and relative prosperity. My good luck goes beyond that: I'm a 1957 baby, the very peak of the boom. Too young to be drafted into the war in Vietnam, too old for the Middle East skirmishing and invading of the last two and a half decades. The most daunting challenges I've confronted in adulthood have been paper cuts, pulled hamstrings, and the odd defriending on Facebook. Remember that Chinese guy who stared down a column of tanks? I once had to stare down a three-hour flight delay.

Prufrock's got nothing on me . . .

Standing in front of the bathroom mirror each morning, we confront the truth. The receding hairline, the hangdog expression, the rounded gut . . . didn't I go to school with that guy? Geez, what happened to him? But the mind's eye sees what it wants to see. The dashing scoundrel. The leading man. The crazy bastard. *Hey look!* Isn't that me chasing Cathy Earnshaw across the moors . . . or urging Ilsa Lund onto the plane . . . or Tarzaning through the homecoming parade, getting even with the squares on the reviewing stand? Well, maybe. But how many of those moments crop up in a lifetime?

Meanwhile, there's a lot of grocery shopping, shoelace threading, and sitting on the train reading hemorrhoid ads. It's in that gap, between our imagined selves and our actual selves, between the heroic and the humdrum, that comedy lies. This is a book about the moments when that gap is yawning.

RIGHT TOOL FOR THE JOB

TURKISH BATH

The memory is simultaneously blurred and seared in my mind. I was seven years old, built like a pond newt, and altogether startled to be spending a Sunday afternoon in 1964 with Morris Goldblatt—who, as a rule, devoted his weekends to solo breakfasts at the Horn & Hardart, marathon poker games at his friends' houses, horse racing at Aqueduct and, after he got home, the Million Dollar Movie on television. For whatever reason, my dad decided that he and I should bond on this particular Sunday. He mentioned the Turkish bath, which meant nothing to me, but he promised that there would be an indoor swimming pool, and afterward, if I wanted, a hot dog with spicy brown mustard, so I pulled on a pair of swimming trunks and a tee shirt and followed him downstairs. Six blocks later—parking was tough in Flushing, Queens—we came to the grimy white Plymouth he was driving that year.

The bathhouse was located in lower Manhattan. I remember a long drive with the sun in my eyes; it must have been around two o'clock when we set out, and we hit patches of traffic. My dad was smoking Camel cigarettes the entire trip, filling the space above the dashboard with a noxious haze, but that seemed normal enough. Then, as we rode across the Brooklyn Bridge, I remember a sudden glimpse of the bleached spires of the Woolworth Building. Now *that* was a sight, a castle fortress jabbing into the cloudless blue sky. What the view must be like from that peak! Once we reached the city, I recall alternating waves of shadow and light bathing the front seat of the car. Then came more driving, very bumpy, more shadow now than light. Then at last we arrived at an underground parking garage, left the car, and walked for two blocks.

I don't remember the facade of the bathhouse itself, only that it didn't look like the kind of place that would have a swimming pool. But I had no reason to think things amiss—or at least no reason until my dad led me through a black metal door, and then down a long echoing hallway and into a dingy gray locker room that smelled of old-man sweat and cooked cabbage, where he told me, in a matter-of-fact tone, as he unbuttoned his trousers, to take off my bathing suit. To which I replied, and this, I am certain, is an exact quote, "Noooooooooooooooooooo!"

He ignored me, but a moment later he thrust a single white towel in my direction, which I pulled at once around my waist, and I determined not to remove it until we were back once again in the locker room, and I could replace it once again with my bathing suit.

"C'mon," he said, looming naked in front of me. "Let's the two of us have a good sweat."

How do I describe what came next? Let me begin with the facts, unembellished. What came next was an elevator ride to the sauna and baths on an upper floor. The elevator was roughly six feet wide by six feet deep. There were perhaps a dozen men, middle-aged and older, crowded into that space. They were all naked.

I was four feet tall.

The sensations of that elevator ride! If I could douse my brain with rubbing alcohol, if I could disinfect the recollection, even at a distance of five decades, I would. Oh, I would in an instant! The undulating cloud of cigar smoke. The baritone laughter from above. The moles and scars. The tufted gray hair. The dimpled, creased and puckered flesh. The crevices.

Whiffs of bowel wherever I turned.

The elevator doors parted, and we stepped out to a smoggy universe of sweating Semites. My dad led me by the left hand into dry-heat rooms and wet-heat rooms, rooms with cracked wooden benches that glistened with film, rooms with hissing, steaming black rocks, rooms with checkerboard tile floors whose central drains were half stopped with furry, seething, coagulating clogs of . . . well, if *ick* were a noun, that would be what the drains were clogged with. With my right hand, as we moved from one room to another, I clung to the white towel cinched around my waist.

I remember my dad grinning down at me and saying, "No one cares about your pee pee, Mark."

Oh, but I did.

We came, in due time, to the swimming pool. It wasn't much, no larger than an average backyard pool, and no deeper than five feet—I gauged this by the fact that the main activity seemed to be arguing rather than swimming. There was a rotating cluster of old men standing in the center of the pool, smoking cigars and cigarettes, thrusting fingers into one another's soggy-haired chests, debating whether Willie Mays was faster than Mickey Mantle *in his prime*, whether Joe Louis was tougher than Jack Dempsey *in his prime*, and whether Sandy Koufax was the greatest Jewish athlete who'd ever lived. The last topic was the most contentious. Several argued for Hank Greenberg, and a lone voice kept bringing up Marty Glickman, whom I did not know at the time but later learned was a world-class sprinter and an All-American football player.

Poolside was where my dad and I spent the next hour. He claimed a lounge chair and began to read the Sunday edition of the *Daily News*; I don't know how he acquired it, whether he'd found it on the chair or borrowed it from a passerby. Once he was distracted, however, I hunkered down. Literally. I squatted on the tile floor, positioned parallel to his head, in a kind of diminished catcher's crouch, still clutching the towel around my waist, averting my eyes from the enormity of his nakedness. (Ham, I would later discover, was cursed in perpetuity for a lack of such courtesy toward his father, Noah.) I can recall vividly the burning in my calves and ankles, but I would not relinquish the position. My dad said to me at one point, "Why don't you go for a swim, for God's sake! Look, there are other boys in the pool!"

Yes, I had noticed them. There were two red-headed boys, probably brothers, wrestling and splashing shamelessly at the shallow end of the pool. The younger one looked roughly my age; the other perhaps two years older. I was in awe of their lack of self-consciousness. Several times, the older allowed the younger to climb onto his shoulders and ride him from one side of the pool to the other. The younger would whoop and yell to call attention to his sudden stature—never mind that his wiener was poking into the back of his brother's head well above the waterline.

"I don't feel like it," I said to my father.

He sighed loudly. "Suit yourself."

Several minutes later, a short, bald, pot-bellied guy with tufted gray hair on his shoulders and back walked over to us. "Hey, Mac," he said, "can you spare part of the paper?"

"Sure thing," my father said. He separated out the sports section and handed it up to the guy.

"You done with it?"

My father nodded.

"What do you think about Koufax?"

"Hell of a pitcher," my father said. "Wish he was still in Brooklyn."

The guy looked down at me. "Maybe you got the next Koufax right there. You play ball, kid?"

I looked straight into his eyes. "Sometimes."

"You pitch?"

"I like the outfield."

"You a runner?"

I nodded. "Yeah."

"You better hope your dick don't get too long."

He and my dad laughed uproariously. I tried to smile at him but felt my face burning.

"He's hanging on to that towel," my dad said.

"Really?"

"He's a funny kid."

"C'mon, kid, loosen up." The guy took a step toward me with his right arm out; I knew at once he intended to snatch the towel from my waist. I frog-jumped several feet to the right and avoided him. He lunged again, but I dodged him and hid behind another lounge chair. He began to laugh again. "You *are* a quick son of a gun, aren't you?"

I managed to smile at him.

"Like a jackrabbit, eh?"

"Yeah," I said.

"Maybe you'll be the next Marty Glickman."

I held my position behind the lounge chair, but I liked the sound of that. I still had no idea who Marty Glickman was except that he was a great athlete, and that he was quick as a jackrabbit . . . and that he and I, come to think of it, had the same initials.

"Maybe," I said.

He smiled knowingly. "You just keep running."

"I will," I said, with conviction.

He turned and walked away. I kept an eye on him until he turned the corner at the end of the pool, and then I exhaled. I glanced from side to side. My dad continued to read his newspaper. The cluster of men in the center of the pool continued their conversation. The two red-headed boys continued wrestling and splashing. No one was paying the slightest attention to me. For the first time since I'd arrived, I felt a measure of relief.

With one hand still on the towel at my waist, I pushed the lounge chair I'd ducked behind next to my father's. Then I climbed up onto it. My eyes were still darting from side to side in case the hairy-shouldered bald guy made another move in my direction. But he'd settled into a lounge chair on the far side of the pool and was occupied with the sports section.

Paradoxically, the fact that the hairy-shouldered bald guy had tried and failed to take away my towel made me feel more secure—as though I'd defended my turf. I *was* too fast for him. He could no more take away my towel than he could Marty Glickman's towel. I sensed the slightest hint of a smile come across my face. As I eased back on the lounge chair, suddenly, I let go of the towel. It was still draped across my waist, but now my hands were free. For several moments, I only sat there, beside my dad. Then, at once, my dad reached over and handed me the comics section from the newspaper. He did this without a word. I took it from him and began to read.

It would be glorious to report that, once I'd finished with the comics, I took another look around, screwed my courage to the sticking place and let the towel slip to the floor . . . that I rose up as Nature had made me, strode to the shallow end of the pool and cannonballed into the ongoing red-headed fracas. But of course that didn't happen. My dad and I sat there for another fifteen minutes, reading the paper, and then he tapped me on the shoulder and told me it was time for dinner.

It would also be glorious to report that the Turkish Bath became a regular retreat for us, a genuine father-son experience. But it turned out to be a one-time deal. I'm sure he felt as though he'd tortured me—which, in a sense, he had.

I remember looking up at him a half hour later, as we ate hot dogs with spicy brown mustard in a Jewish delicatessen, rating him against the collection of old naked guys I'd seen that afternoon, and thinking: *I could've done worse for a father.*

MANHOOD, PART ONE

During the second week of May in 1970, two weeks before my bar mitzvah, I wet my pants. It happened during seventh-grade social studies class. I had been rocking back and forth at my desk, dreading a quiz on India and Pakistan that I hadn't studied for, when I suddenly realized I was soggy.

The first thing I did was . . . nothing. I sat motionless as the warm soak issued out from my groin. I could feel it running in rivulets in my underwear. After the initial sensation wore off, sheer disbelief set in. I hadn't wet myself since—well, I'd never wet myself. Or at least I hadn't wet myself since I was in diapers and thus dressed for the occasion.

How could it have happened? I was a *seventh grader*, for Christ's sake! a bar mitzvah boy within the month! And I'd just wet myself? None of my peers had peed their pants since the dawn of grammar school, or at least not to my knowledge, and until that moment I'd figured that that particular form of classroom theater had been laid to rest. The last classmate I could recall shooting the rapids was Georgia, a third grader on whom I had a minor crush, who burst into tears and bolted from the classroom—the backside of her bright pink dress telling the sordid tale as she fled.

Even then, I remember thinking: *How does that happen?*

I mean, it wasn't as if the procedure for requesting a bathroom break was difficult to master. You raised your hand. The teacher called on you. You said, "May I go to the bathroom?" You did *not* say, "*Can* I go to the bathroom?" The distinction was crucial, according to my mom. The question "*Can* I go to the bathroom?" meant *Does my thingamajig work?* Whereas the question "*May* I go to the bathroom?" meant *Am I permitted to leave the room and do what I need to do?*

The difference between *may* and *can*, my mom said, might not seem like a big deal right now, but it was the difference between good manners and no manners. She told me to mark her words.

So I marked her words.

In any event, getting to the bathroom in time to do your business wasn't exactly like working a slide rule. You raised your hand. The teacher called on you. Even if you slipped and said *can* instead of *may*, the teacher still nodded and let you go. Unless the need arose instantaneously—which seemed, in my experience, highly unlikely—how could you screw it up?

Yet here I was, two weeks from stepping up to the podium in Temple Gates of Prayer, two weeks from leading the congregation through a reading of the *haftarah*, here I was, in seventh-grade social studies, suddenly awash in my Fruit of the Looms.

Still, I didn't panic.

Taking stock of the predicament, I quickly realized that I'd caught a couple of breaks. The first was the fifteen-minute quiz that the teacher, Mr. Roth, was handing out at that very moment. The quiz I had no chance to pass. Things dry out in fifteen minutes, I told myself. If I sat still, with my legs slightly parted, and let nature go to work, I might be able to stand up at the end and walk my quiz sheet to the front of the room without urine trickling down the legs of my pants.

The second break I caught was the pants themselves. The material was light cotton, which was bad, but the color was olive green—which would conceal, to a certain extent, the ground-zero stain that was no doubt gathering into a Rorschach pattern below my belt buckle. (I didn't dare slide back my seat to look.) If I could just get to the front desk, turn in my quiz, then get back to my seat without incident, I'd have another hour to recess until I had to rise from my desk again.

I might pull this off, I thought.

Mr. Roth dropped the mimeographed quiz on the desk in front of me and did not break stride. The smell of flop sweat was strong on him; it was a very grown-up smell, tinged with cigarette smoke. I did not touch the quiz, however, until he was back in front of the room. He sat on the edge of his metal desk, looked down his horn-rimmed glasses at the class, and said, "You may begin."

The sound of papers flipping over filled the air, and I exhaled. My situation, for the time being, was the last thing anyone would notice. I made a cursory show of skimming down the quiz. Again, there was no chance I was going to pass; I hadn't read the assigned textbook chapter because the weather had warmed up the week before, and I'd played softball and roundup tag to exhaustion each night since. One quiz question caught my eye, however: "How is the population estimated in the rural towns and villages in India?"

I picked up my pencil and wrote in the provided space: "One little, two little, three little Indians."

As the minutes rolled past, I was feeling more and more hopeful about my prospects. I was still damp but by no means drenched. I took a casual glance around the room. None of the other students were paying the slightest attention to what I was doing. They were intent on the quiz. Now, I thought, would be a good time to slide back my chair, ever so slightly, and survey the damage.

I'd moved less than an inch when I heard Mr. Roth's voice. "Mr. Goldblatt?"

"Yes?" I muttered.

Suddenly, I could feel every eye in the classroom trained on me.

"Are you cheating, Mr. Goldblatt?"

I shook my head vehemently. "No."

"Then why are you looking down?"

"I . . . I . . ."

He hopped off his desk and hustled up the aisle in my direction. The flop sweat and cigarette smell engulfed me; I looked up at him in desperation and confusion. "Stand up, Mr. Goldblatt."

"I wasn't cheating, Mr. Roth."

"Stand up!"

"But I wasn't—"

"I'm asking you for the last time."

Braced for a wave of laughter, and the end of life as I knew it, I shut my eyes, slid back my chair, and stood up.

There was no reaction. Not a sound.

I heard Mr. Roth say, "I *saw* you cheating, Mr. Goldblatt."

I opened my eyes. "I swear I wasn't cheating, Mr. Roth."

"Empty your pockets."

"What?"

"You heard me, Mr. Goldblatt."

I reached into the right-front pocket of my pants, anticipating its contents would be thoroughly marinated, or at least noticeably moist, but miraculously came out with a bone-dry handkerchief and three nickels. I set the handkerchief and nickels down on the desk, then looked back up at Mr. Roth.

"Now the other pockets . . ."

"There's nothing in the other pockets, Mr. Roth."

"Humor me."

I pulled my left-front pocket inside out, then both back pockets. There was not a trace of the earlier flood. I smiled up at him. "I told you."

He grabbed me by the waist and spun me around, then patted me down, front and back. He opened up the top of the desk and rifled through the storage compartment. Then he got down on his knees and checked the floor.

He found nothing.

"All right, Mr. Goldblatt. Sit down . . . but know that I've got my eye on you."

"Yes, Mr. Roth."

"I'm watching you like a hawk."

"Yes, Mr. Roth."

"The rest of you," he called, "get back to your quizzes!"

With that, the class went back to work, and I exhaled.

How could it have happened? I *knew* I'd wet my pants. There was no doubt in my mind. It hadn't been a hallucination. I'd felt it, not *thought* that I'd felt it. But how could it have dried so fast? The universe worked according to certain laws; I'd learned that in general science class. My pants *were* wet, then *were not* wet. Maybe there was a God, I thought. Maybe He'd looked down on me and cut me slack because of the whole bar mitzvah thing.

I filled in several more answers on the quiz . . . took wild guesses at names and dates and places; if God had solved one problem for me, maybe he'd solve the rest. Maybe I had a get-out-of-jail-free card good through my bar mitzvah. As the fifteen-minute time limit came to a close, I folded the quiz sheet in half and walked it up to the front desk. Mr. Roth narrowed his eyes at me as he took it from my hand, but he said nothing more.

When recess arrived an hour later, I made a beeline for the boy's bathroom, locked myself in a stall, and surveyed the accident scene. There was no urine; there was a slight dampness at the front of my underwear, centered at the flap, but the warm rivulets I'd felt against my skin were gone. Could the cotton be that absorbent? I pulled up my pants and left the stall without a rational explanation. For the rest of the afternoon, I put the incident from my mind.

As I rode the bus home from school later that afternoon, however, it began to nag at me again. What had happened? I skipped the Fig Newtons and Kool-Aid my mom had laid out on the kitchen table and motored straight to the bathroom. There, under the strong overhead light, I discovered a curious phenomenon I'd missed in the stall at school. There were dried flecks of what appeared to be Elmer's glue on the inside flap of my underwear; on closer examination, there were flecks on my skin as well. How could glue have gotten in my underwear? I did have a plastic tube in the storage compartment of my desk, but I hadn't used it for weeks.

The entire incident, from start to finish, seemed inexplicable. I told no one, of course; I wasn't about to announce that I'd wet my pants. I couldn't dwell on it anyway. I had Hebrew passages to memorize.

My poor performance on the India and Pakistan quiz—I scored a fifty-one—had the paradoxical effect of convincing Mr. Roth that I *hadn't* cheated . . . and that he'd shamed me in front of the class without cause. It turned out he had also asked a couple of notorious squealers whether they'd noticed me with a crib sheet, and one of them had speculated that I might have been studying for my bar mitzvah rather than cheating on the quiz. Whatever the case, Mr. Roth pulled me aside the following morning and apologized; he told me that he'd laughed at the "one little, two little, three little Indians" joke, and wished me good luck at temple.

As I was about to turn and walk away, he clasped my shoulder and added, "It's your big moment. Don't screw it up."

Until he spoke those words, the thought that I could screw up my *haftarah* reading had never crossed my mind. Sure, I'd be nervous; sure, I might get the intonations wrong. But *screw it up outright*? Freeze at the podium? It wasn't an outcome I'd ever considered. The more I thought about it, though, the more real the possibility became. I had been working with the original Hebrew texts, but between the lines I'd scribbled full English transliterations—so that even if I blanked on the right-to-left characters, I could fall back on the left-to-right nonsense syllables in my own handwriting. That was my safety net. But by the time I got home, Mr. Roth's words were ringing inside my head. The four pages of my *haftarah* suddenly looked like a blur of scratches and doodles, like something you'd find on an abandoned Etch A Sketch. How could a human being stand up in front of his relatives and friends and make sense of *that*?

Starting at that moment, and for the next two weeks, I was a nervous wreck. I tried to memorize the entire four pages, to rehearse the sounds in my head again and again so that I no longer had to look at the Hebrew or the transliteration—but the more I tried to memorize, the less I seemed to remember. I woke up three days before the event and could not begin.

Literally, I could not recall the first word.

What I *could* recall, in more and more vivid detail, were bar mitzvah calamities I'd witnessed. Bad things happened at that podium. The year before, for instance, Eric, a kid from down the block, had walked up to the podium, stared down at the crowded pews, opened his mouth—and nothing came out. Dead silence. For a full minute, an eon of a minute, there was dead silence . . . punctuated, after fifteen seconds, by nervous coughs and whispers from the congregation, until at long last the rabbi stepped forward, put his arm around Eric's shoulders, and led him through his entire *haftarah*, three halting Hebrew words at a time.

Then there was Asher, a brainiac I'd known since second grade, who ascended the stage with noticeable confidence and began, at once, to sweat. Beads of sweat formed across his forehead and glistened in the hot lights of the temple stage. They trickled into his eyes one by one, blinding him to the text, until the rabbi stepped forward with a handful of Kleenex. Asher finished his *haftarah* with his curly brown hair matted to his scalp, his starched pink collar soaked through, mopping his brow like Louis Armstrong after a long trumpet solo.

Then, of course, there were the urban legends, twice-told tales of friends of friends who took to the podium and fainted. Or wept. Or vomited.

Or wet their pants.

So it came to pass that on the twenty-second day of the ninth month of the year 5730—that's May 28, 1970, if you're playing along at home—a mere forty-eight hours before I was set to become a man, with random sacred words swirling around in my brain, and with images of imminent humiliation roiling my bowels, I awakened just after sunrise . . . having wet my bed.

I lurched upright to a sitting position and muttered, "Oh no!"

But I could feel the truth gathering inside my pajamas, pooling in my lap, running down my right thigh, and puddling underneath me. I'd wet my bed, through my pajamas, and I had no doubt, none whatsoever, that I was going to wet myself again at the podium as I recited my *haftarah*.

I was doomed.

When I pulled back the covers and pulled down my pajama pants, however, I found not urine but a milky white liquid coagulating on and around me. Terrifyingly, it was still dribbling from the aperture of my penis.

Now, at once, the bar mitzvah was the least of my worries: I wasn't doomed . . . *I was dying.*

Two courses of action suggested themselves. 1) Wake up my parents and tell them what had happened; 2) Wait a couple of hours and tell my best friend, Lonnie. After several moments of deliberation, I chose Lonnie because I wanted him to say nice things about me at my funeral, and I knew he'd feel slighted if I turned first to my parents—who *had* to say nice things about me regardless.

Lonnie was always the last kid to line up for the school bus, rolling out of his house a half minute before the bus itself rolled up Parsons Boulevard. That was part of his mystique. He was a year older than I was and the coolest kid I knew, the coolest kid anyone I knew knew, and every night, when I hit my knees and laid me down to sleep, I thanked God that Lonnie and I had become friends long before either of us had a clear grasp of the concept of *cool*. Had we met afterward, he wouldn't have given me the time of day.

Lonnie was still yawning as I dragged him by the sleeve to the back of the bus, to the very last pair of seats, and pinky-swore him to secrecy. Then I told him that I was dying, and he looked at me with extreme skepticism, so I told him the entire sordid history, starting with me wetting my pants in social studies class and ending with me wetting my bed that morning.

As I came to the end, he began to laugh.

"It's not funny!" I whispered.

"You don't even know how funny it is."

"It's funny that I'm dying?"

"You're not dying. You're not even sick."

"How do you know?"

"You *jerked off*. That's all that happened."

"I did not!"

"You did too. You jerked off."

"No way!"

"Then you tell me. What else could it be?"

"Not that," I said.

He looked at me quizzically for a split second. Then a sudden recognition came to face. "You don't know what I'm talking about, do you?"

"Yes, I do—"

"You don't know what *jerking off* means."

"I know what it means!"

"All right, what does it mean?"

I tried to hold a look of indignation. But it was no use. He had me dead to rights. I'd heard the phrase hundreds of times; I'd heard it used as a verb and as a noun. Hell, I'd even used it myself. But until that moment, I thought it had to do with wasting time. As in: *That guy's just sitting at home, jerking off . . . what a jerk-off!*

Clearly, there was another definition.

I lowered my eyes. "Okay, I don't know what it means."

"I knew it!"

I shushed him. "C'mon, just tell me."

His voice dropped. "Look, it's nothing to be ashamed of."

"I'm not ashamed—"

"I don't get why you didn't just ask me in the first place."

"What difference does it make?" I said. "I'm asking now."

He leaned back. "Well, it means . . . you know, *jerking off*."

"Yes—"

"It means getting a boner and jerking off."

"Okay."

"Do you know what a *boner* is?"

I nodded—which was the truth.

"When you get a boner, you jerk off. Not all the time, but sometimes. It's normal."

"So you think that's what happened?"

"No, I'm *sure* that's what happened."

"How do I keep it from happening again?"

"Why would you want to do that?" he said. "Didn't it feel good?"

"No!"

"Don't you want to *do it*?"

"Sure, I do," I said, ashamed to admit he'd lost me again.

"Then, there you go."

"What does one thing have to do with the other?"

Lonnie sighed. "You still don't know what we're talking about."

"I do so!"

He shook his head. "Look, are we friends or not?"

"Sure we are."

"Then why are you lying to me?"

That got to me. "I don't . . . it's just that—"

"What?"

"You're right," I said. "I don't know what we're talking about."

The school bus slowed to a stop at a traffic light. Between that traffic light and the next one, a space of perhaps three minutes, Lonnie explained the facts of life. There were no metaphors. No talk of love or connectedness or commitment. Neither a bird nor a bee made a cameo appearance in his disquisition. He used blunt language and occasional hand gestures.

He told me *what went where.*

By the end of his talk, I had forgotten that I was dying. I had forgotten that I had a *haftarah* to learn and recite, that my relatives and friends were going to gather in the temple on Saturday, the day after tomorrow, to witness my bar mitzvah. The totality of what I felt, the totality of thoughts and emotions, the totality of my consciousness at that moment, was revulsion.

I stared down between my legs. "I'm not doing that. Not ever."

"Sure, you will," Lonnie said. "Everybody does it. It's natural."

"No way . . . no way."

"Your parents did it. Your mom and dad."

"Oh, come on!"

"How do you think you got here?" he said.

"I don't know."

"Your parents did it. Their parents did it. Their parents' parents did it. Their parents' parents' parents' did it, going all the way back to Adam and Eve. That's how the world works."

I lifted my eyes up to meet his. "Are you sure?"

"I'm sure."

"Who told you?"

"My dad told me some. The rest I figured out for myself."

"You're okay with it?"

"Not at first," he said. "I was like you. I thought about my mom and dad doing it, and I thought *no way*. That's what everybody thinks at first. But the more you think about it, the more sense it makes. Just think about how things fit together. It's like when you're doing a puzzle. You know when it's right because the pieces just fit . . ." Each sentence he spoke felt like a punch to the gut. The sounds of the words themselves were nauseating. I wanted him to stop, but I didn't know how to ask. My head sank lower and lower until at last he interrupted himself and said, "You look like you're going to puke."

I glanced up. "I've just got a bad taste in my mouth."

"You're not going to puke, are you?"

"No, it's nothing like that," I said.

"It's tough the first time you hear it. But then it's not so bad. Trust me."

I wanted to trust him. I *did* trust him. That's what was making it worse.

Lonnie and I parted company as soon as the bus pulled up in front of the school. He was a grade ahead of me and had a different set of friends at school. He trotted off to meet them at the entrance of the schoolyard, and I went straight to my homeroom. I sat down at my desk and began scanning the room from side to side, wondering which of my classmates, shuffling through their papers, getting their assignments in order, knew the ugly truth. It *couldn't* be that many, I decided. Maybe Donald and Sherm . . . they were tall. Maybe Hector too because he spoke Spanish. Asher was another possibility, even though he'd sweated through his bar mitzvah suit, because he was a brainiac. But none of the girls knew. I was certain of that.

I mean: *If the girls knew, how could they bear to sit next to the boys?*

I tried to tough it out once class began but lasted only until lunch. That was when I told Mr. Roth that I felt sick to my stomach—which was true. I knew, of course, that he'd write it off to pre-bar mitzvah jitters. He clasped me by the shoulder and winked at me. He smelled, as always, of flop sweat and cigarette smoke. Right then, all I could think about was Mr. Roth *doing it.*

My mom drove to school and picked me up at the nurse's office. Riding home, I thought about her doing it with my dad. Then, for one horrible moment, I thought about her doing it with Mr. Roth.

"Are you worried about Saturday morning, honey?"

I stared out the passenger side window. "I guess."

"There's nothing to worry about. You'll do fine."

"I guess."

"Whatever happens, you know that I'm very proud of you. Your father is too."

I thought: *They probably talk about how proud they are while they're doing it.*

I holed up in my room once I got home, alternating between taking short naps and watching *The Three Stooges* and *Gilligan's Island* on a portable black and white Zenith television. My mom knocked on the door after sunset and handed me a peanut butter sandwich and a glass of grape juice. That was the only human contact I had. I don't remember whether I dreamed that night, but I woke up Friday morning and decided to skip school. I called the decision out to my mom through the closed door.

I gave her no reason; she didn't ask for one.

That entire Friday I spent in front of the Zenith, with the sound turned down to an inaudible level, not so much watching it as wallowing in its rays. At one point, I brought over my *haftarah* from the desk, set it on my lap and tried to concentrate on it, but my mind kept wandering back to Ricochet Rabbit and his partner, Droop-a-long. *Doing it.* If I screwed up my bar mitzvah, I thought, so what?

The last thought I had before falling asleep on Friday night, the last words I spoke, in lieu of my prayers, were: *So what?*

Of course, I didn't screw up my bar mitzvah the following morning. I stepped up to the stage in the temple in my blue suit and tie, looked out at the congregation from behind the podium, and didn't miss a single word, a single syllable, a single accent. I didn't glance once at my *haftarah*, neither the original text nor the transliteration. I had the thing memorized. The Hebrew sounds flowed out of me as though I knew what they meant, as though I were thinking holy thoughts and giving them voice rather than staring down at my parents in the front row, noticing them holding hands and imagining them *doing it.*

Afterward, the rabbi stepped forward and shook my hand. He spoke to me in front of the congregation for several minutes; the only words I can recall were, "The Lord works in mysterious ways."

THE DELVECCHIO BEATDOWN

Mike Delvecchio was the toughest kid in ninth grade at Edward Bleeker Junior High School. I can still see him strutting across the asphalt of the school yard, a box of Lucky Strikes peeking out from his rolled-up right sleeve, an entourage of demi-thugs trailing in his wake. He was built like a fire hydrant, and he seemed to have been formed from the knuckles outward, his tight face, dense neck, and veined forearms mere secondary expressions of his balled-up right fist.

That balled-up right fist . . . the collective nightmares of the male half of the entire ninth grade were realized in that fist. Bravado counts for much among pubescent boys, but, with respect to Mike Delvecchio, common sense prevailed. If you ever caused him offense, the question was not whether to run, but in what direction to run, for how long, and, oh, by the way, did the Witness Relocation Program accept minors?

With respect to Mike Delvecchio, I repeat, common sense prevailed . . . with the lone exception of Phillip Spindler. I suspect there's a Phillip Spindler in everybody's junior high school experience. The kid who never got with the program, who wouldn't eat licorice because it was sold unwrapped, who wouldn't join the recess game of tag until dutifully limbering up, who would trade his Scooter Pie for a second orange during cold and flu season. The Phillip Spindler I remember was Bic-pen thin, his glasses thick as Petri dishes, and he always toted a shiny black attaché case. It was the attaché case, amid an ocean of knapsacks, that caught Mike Delvecchio's eye one afternoon after school. He came up behind Phillip Spindler and "snagged" it to the pavement. The thing broke open, its metal snaps mangled, and Phillip Spindler's loose papers swirled across the suburban lawns of Whitestone.

"Psych!" Mike Delvecchio cried.

He and his gang broke into uproarious laughter.

Phillip Spindler didn't scramble to retrieve the papers. He didn't move. He faced Mike Delvecchio. His eyes narrowed, his lower lip quivering with anger.

"You wanna make somethin' of it?" Mike Delvecchio asked.

Phillip Spindler didn't respond. He continued to stand motionless.

The standoff lasted another five seconds until, at last, Mike Delvecchio shouted, "Double psych!" Then he turned and walked off. His gang shot Phillip Spindler a few nasty glares, then followed.

That should've ended the story. It didn't, because childhood is never kind to the Phillip Spindlers of the world. He trudged home that afternoon, his ruined attaché case hugged to his chest, and told his father what had happened. Whereupon his father advised him that the only way to deal with a bully was to stand up to him. It was just the kind of advice that worked on *Father Knows Best, Leave It to Beaver*, and *Andy Griffith*. The trouble, of course, was that Mike Delvecchio never watched those shows. He spent his evenings in the alley smoking Lucky Strikes.

The following morning, before our homeroom teacher walked in, Phillip Spindler announced that he was going to stand up to Mike Delvecchio. He used the exact words. *Stand up*. Several of us tried to talk him out of it. But he was determined. He quoted his father to us, and we shook our heads.

By three o'clock, word had reached Mike Delvecchio that some geek from the *gifted* class intended to stand up to him. He showed up at the appointed intersection first, before Phillip Spindler, pounding his clenched right fist into the palm of his left hand. He shadow-boxed as he waited for his challenger to appear; the curiosity on his face was evident. When he saw who it was, a look of disappointment, almost remorse, came over him. He hadn't expected the kid with the Petri dish glasses from the previous afternoon. Still, he handed his Lucky Strikes to one of his flunkies and strode up to Phillip Spindler. He jabbed his forefinger hard into Phillip Spindler's chest and said, "You get the first shot."

Phillip Spindler turned around, handed his glasses to the nearest bystander, who happened to be me, and then, in a single motion, wheeled around and punched Mike Delvecchio right in the stomach.

There was a loud gasp . . .

It came from the crowd of onlookers.

The punch had no effect whatsoever on Mike Delvecchio.

The pummeling he gave Phillip Spindler that afternoon lasted several minutes, and, in the end, Mike Delvecchio didn't seem to take much pleasure in it. He went strictly by the numbers: He flung Phillip Spindler to the ground, banged his head on the sidewalk, split his lower lip, blackened his right eye. But there was none of the usual Delvecchio panache, no signature, like the time he straddled Kenneth Conway's chest and farted in his face.

Later, as four of us struggled to extricate Phillip Spindler from the sticker bushes where Mike Delvecchio had deposited him, I began to feel a grudging admiration for him, an admiration that bordered on envy; the scariest thing that could happen had happened, and now it was over, and he had lived through it. There seemed indeed an odd dignity about Phillip Spindler at that moment, about the way he pushed his glasses back onto his head, wincing slightly as they came to rest on his swollen cheekbones. Several weeks later, I thought of him in English class as I was reading the closing passage of *The Red Badge of Courage*: "He had been to touch the great death, and found that, after all, it was but the great death."

Maybe in the greater scheme of things, Mike Delvecchio never quite ranked with "the great death." But the truth about ninth grade is that the greater scheme of things has not yet begun to register. For that year, at least, the guy couldn't have been scarier if he'd carried a sickle.

MANHOOD, PART TWO

The closest I ever came to a summer of '42 was the summer of '73—a summer I spent at Rosmarins bungalow colony in the Catskill Mountains of New York. My family had taken a bungalow there for several years, but that summer, the summer I turned sixteen, they decided to stay in the city. To my astonishment, however, they let me rent a bungalow with another boy, Perry, whom I'd gotten to know during past summers at Rosmarins. It was such a half-baked plan—two sixteen-year-olds, left alone, with their own bungalow, for the entire summer—that neither Perry nor I ever believed our parents would go for it; I recall laughing when he first floated the idea over the phone. But go for it our parents did, and then they convinced Old Man Rosmarin, the kind-hearted owner of colony, to stick his neck out. He agreed to rent us the least popular bungalow on the colony; it was set at the base of a steep hill, at the edge of a dense woods. He also agreed to defray part of the expense by hiring us as junior counselors in his day camp. He went along with the idea because he'd known both of us for years and knew we were nice boys. Which we were.

Until that summer.

Here's the sum of what I knew about human sexuality on Memorial Day, 1973: *what went where*. I knew the proper names for the *what* and the *where*, as well as several of the coarser monosyllabic variants. I knew that if the man's *what* engaged the woman's *where* under the right conditions, a baby was made. That was about it. Perry, it turned out, knew more. Not all of what he knew was accurate, but in our late-night conversations that first week in the bungalow we talked a lot of baseball: He explained what getting to first, second, and third bases meant, what non-verbal cues to watch for at each stage, and under what conditions it would be possible to slide home. I was grateful for the analogy. I was appalled by the acts he was describing.

Soon enough, Perry was putting theory into practice. He had a leg up in that he looked like a young Peter Noone, which, along with the fact that he now had a bachelor's pad at his disposal, proved irresistible to colony girls elsewhere inhibited by the watchful gaze of one another's moms. By the end of our third week in the bungalow, Perry was juggling three girlfriends and was commandeering the bedroom for hours at a stretch.

I, meanwhile, was torn. Strive as I might to give Perry privacy, to sequester myself at the critical moment on the screened-in porch at the front of the bungalow, I could not avoid the accidents of his performances—the sights and sounds, as well as the percussive thudding of bed against wall. I was the odd guy out. That experience, according to every low-, medium-, and high-budget teen film ever made, should've been alternately arousing and maddening. Instead, it was dispiriting and depressing. Perry's graphic accounts after the fact did nothing but diminish my desire to follow his lead.

Except for Inger Stevens, I might have taken a vow of chastity.

There is a fair chance that a reader in the second decade of the twenty-first century will not recognize the name Inger Stevens. (There is a fair chance such a reader will have skimmed over earlier references to *Summer of '42* and Peter Noone, come to think of it.) She was a Swedish-American actress often remembered, if she is remembered at all, as the wholesome title character in a TV series called *The Farmer's Daughter*, which ran from 1963 to 1966. I seem to recall watching the show once or twice, maybe in reruns, and noticing only that she was exceptionally pretty. The more lasting impression Inger Stevens made on me came from the racy (for that era) 1967 movie *A Guide for the Married Man*, in which she played the wife of a philandering husband played by Walter Matthau. I saw the movie in an edited-for-television version around 1970—right about the time puberty had begun working its mischief. The plot is irrelevant. What matters is a single scene: Inger Stevens, in white leotard, exercising on a bed. She is on her back, hoisting her butt in the air, bicycling her legs. Then she's on all fours, doing leg lifts, her blond hair flying backward. Afterward, as Matthau watches, she strips off the leotard. The camera closes in on her bare back.. . . It is not an exaggeration to say that that scene changed my life. (Morbid aside: Right about the time Inger Stevens was yanking me abruptly from boyhood to manhood, she was ingesting a lethal overdose of narcotics. My first sexual crush was likely posthumous.) Whatever thoughts I had from that moment on of a *what* and a *where* co-joined involved Inger Stevens.

However disconcerting Perry's bungalow trysts might have been, they were always counterbalanced by the image of Inger Stevens, working up a sweat, in that white leotard, on that quilted bed.

Enter into the equation a junior counselor named Kristyn. New to Rosmarins that summer, she was slender, with light blue eyes, high cheekbones, long blond hair, and a delicate button of a nose—that last, a decided rarity among the second- and third-generation Ashkenazi honkers that prevailed at the colony. I was also drawn to the exotic *y* in her name, which seemed like the bendy kind of vowel Inger Stevens would have had in her name, except that she didn't.

I confessed my feelings for Kristyn to Perry. It was a strategic move, since I feared she might otherwise wind up another of his conquests. He scouted her and gave me a heartfelt thumbs-up. What remained was to win her affections—no minor task, since she seemed to have no clue of my presence at the bungalow colony, or on the planet. Still, Perry and I decided that I should woo her, because he'd begun to feel bad about hogging the bedroom, and it was selfish of me to put him in that position. The thought of striking up a conversation with her terrified me, but he told me not to worry. "They can smell fear," he said. Besides, all I had to do was sit next to her during the Saturday-night movie at the clubhouse, and then, at exactly the right moment, slip my arm around her shoulders; nature would do the rest. But how would I know when the moment was exactly right? Perry shushed me. "Trust your instincts," he said.

The film at the clubhouse that weekend was *The Heartbreak Kid*, in which Cybill Shepherd stars as, well, Inger Stevens. Perry had enlisted a half dozen buddies of ours in the cause, and the group of them ran a flanking maneuver worthy of General George Patton, peeling away members of Kristyn's she-pack one by one, to ensure that there would be a seat available beside her. She did not seem fazed by my sudden appearance on her left, nor by the perfect boy-girl-boy-girl sequence that materialized in defiance of the law of averages on her right, as if to underscore the fact that she and I were together.

"Hi," I said.

She looked at me in a quizzical way, then sighed and settled back into her wooden folding chair. The fact that she didn't stand up and walk out, I interpreted as tacit consent. Still without a word, she turned her attention to the screen as the movie projector began to whir.

It was roughly a half hour into the movie, around the time Cybill Shepherd makes her first appearance, that I slipped my right arm over Kristyn's shoulders. There was no pretense to the gesture, no fake yawn or coincidental stretch across the back of her chair. My instinct told me that the moment was right, so I acted. To my amazement, she rested her head at once on my right shoulder. Instinctively, again, I kissed the top of her head, and then rested my right cheek against her hair.

For the next hour and a half, I did not move my right arm, she did not move her head from my right shoulder, and I did not move my right cheek from her hair. Rodin couldn't have sculpted us more static. I lost all sensation from my right pectoral muscle to the fingertips of my right hand. But I did not move, not until the end credits began to roll, and I felt her head rise against my right cheek. I sat up and let my right arm fall behind her chair. It felt like dead meat. As I was flexing my jaw, which also was numb, I sensed her eyes watching me under the darkness. I turned to face her, and then at once our lips came together. She had initiated the kiss. It was very soft and very dry and without emotion. It lasted for perhaps five seconds and ended as the lights in the clubhouse came up. For a split second, however, the lights were on, and we were still kissing.

I felt certain Perry had noticed.

Tingling had returned to my right arm as we filed out of the clubhouse. It occurred to me to take her hand, but we were not quite side by side going up the center aisle; she was just out of reach. By the time we were on the path to the bungalows, our not-holding-hands seemed established. Mind you, except for that initial *hi* of mine, we still hadn't spoken to one another.

Several minutes later, we stood in front of her parents' bungalow. She turned toward me and smiled in a mysterious way. Her first words to me were, "I don't know your name."

"It's Mark," I said.

"Do you know my name?"

"Yes."

"Thanks for the movie."

"It was free."

"I know that," she said.

"I didn't *pay* for you."

She shook her head. I leaned forward to kiss her, but she turned and walked inside.

"You're an idiot," Perry said, after I told him what had happened. The two of us were sitting on the porch, sipping cans of discount cola, watching fireflies flitting through the darkness. Mosquitoes were buzzing invisibly just beyond the screen windows; every so often one of them would crash into one of the screens, driven mad by the blaze of lights within.

"I got to first base," I said, sheepishly.

"That's as far as you're *going* to get."

"How can you possibly know that?"

But of course Perry was right. Kristyn jogged up to me as I was wrangling seven-year-old campers the following Monday and told me that she wanted to break up. As I formulated a counterargument, she turned and jogged off, her blond hair streaming behind her. That was that. We were done in under twenty-five words. I was left stranded on first base.

Second base, or thereabouts, would come three weeks later in the form of a girl named Candy. Unlike Kristyn, who flitted in and out of my thoughts like a firefly, Candy was a familiar fixture in my psychic landscape. We had known one another for eight years—half of our lives—going back to a previous bungalow colony. The first time I'd laid eyes on her, she was holding a sunflower and skipping back and forth in front of her parents' bungalow. Literally, skipping. She was angelic-faced, her skin pale to the point of translucence, with short brown hair and sad brown eyes, and she gave me a pain in the heart. Again, literally: I remember holding my chest and watching her. I'd dreamed of taking her hand when we were eight, of kissing her on the lips when we were ten, of marrying her when we were twelve. But then, the summer we turned thirteen, something happened to her. She began to crack up. She'd mutter to herself and weep for no reason and wear black dresses to teen bowling nights. By the time I knew *what went where*, the only feelings I had for Candy were bewilderment and pity.

Not that she lacked male attention. Puberty had hit her in a spectacular way. Her chest developed in defiance of architectural likelihood, and her sad brown eyes, by the summer of '73, had acquired a lunatic disorientation that seemed to smolder with sexual promise. Before the term was coined, she was a *hot mess*. I remember one kid named Robbie watching her walk past us in a low-cut evening gown, then holding out his hands to indicate the shape of her breasts, and muttering, "Succulent." It was the wettest, dirtiest word I'd ever heard.

Candy had suitors galore, and with the slightest nod of interest, she could have had her pick of junior and senior counselors—and perhaps even a few of the wayward husbands on the colony. But as far as I knew, she nodded at no one. She roamed the colony grounds in a world of her own, too old to attend the camp, too distracted to work as a counselor, oblivious to the stares and whispers and occasional snickers that followed her.

I don't think I ever made a conscious decision to approach her. But the two of us crossed paths late one afternoon while I was walking home from camp. Candy had on a blue flower-print sundress—a grudging acknowledgment of the heat and humidity of the first week in August as well as a noticeable break from her usual Vampirella wardrobe. The dress was wildly out of synch with the tank tops and shorts favored by teenage girls at Rosmarins, but at least it made her seem less lost.

She looked up, and our eyes locked. Still, she would have walked past me without a word had I not caught her by the left arm. She stopped and faced me; her gaze turned into a stare. There was no alarm in her expression, just curiosity of a disproportionately intense kind.

"I only wanted to say hello," I managed.

"Is that it?"

"Are you all right, Candy?"

"Why would you ask me that question?"

"I don't know. You don't seem all right."

"Why?"

"You don't seem like yourself," I said.

"Who do I seem like?"

"I don't know."

"Do you know who I am?" she asked.

"Yes, I do. Do you know who I am?"

"You're a boy I used to know."

"You still know me."

She only smiled at the thought.

"Do you want to take a walk?" I said.

"Where?"

"You've never seen my bungalow."

"Why do you call it that?"

"Because that's what it is," I said.

"Why do you say it's *yours*?"

"Because it is. For the summer."

"Nothing is yours *for the summer*. Either it's yours or it's not yours."

I shook my head. "Candy, do you want to see my bungalow or not?"

She smiled. "If you want to show it to me."

"I do."

I put out my hand, and she took it. It was a quarter-mile walk along the main road and then down the steep grassy incline to the bungalow.

Her steps were tentative; she had on red flip-flops, not her usual black heels, and blisters had formed where the plastic strap caught her skin. She would laugh from time to time as we walked, for no reason that I could discern, then squeeze my hand as if to ascertain its reality. As the bungalow came into sight, I stopped abruptly—overcome with guilt at what I had in mind. Her eyes bore in on mine again. "What now?"

"Candy, I'm not sure—"

"Don't you want to show me *your* bungalow?"

"Stop saying it like that."

She let go of my hand and ran down the hill to the bungalow door. Her entire torso seemed to liquefy as she gained speed; her breasts, even observed at an angle from behind, were pendulous and uncontrollable. Their effect was hypnotic and nauseating. I followed several steps after her, wishing our paths had never crossed. She called back, "Is the door locked?"

"No," I said.

She opened the door and disappeared inside.

I expected to find her on the porch, or perhaps in the kitchen, but she had bypassed both and gone straight to the bedroom. I found her sitting on the edge of my bed, staring at me with a blank expression. She was either looking past me or through me; I couldn't tell which. After several seconds, she said, "Well?"

"Do you want a soda?" I said.

She shook her head, then patted the mattress next to her. She wanted me to sit down. I didn't know what else to do, so I sat down. For several more seconds, there was an equilibrium between us. We sat rigidly, inches apart, at the edge of the bed. Then, at once, she took my right hand and slipped it inside her sundress and onto her left breast. I neither resisted nor cooperated. It was her will, her doing. My hand lay lifelessly on her breast. We were both looking down at the event as though it were an abstraction, a random juxtaposition of hand and breast that involved neither of us. Out of desperation, I leaned in and kissed her on the mouth. I could feel her arousal against my palm. Then I felt her arms slide around my neck.

There are a few moments that define you as a person, that cut to the core of who you are, moments in which you discover lines you will and won't cross. This was the first one for me: I would fondle the breast of a girl who wasn't in her right mind . . . but that was as far as I would go. I figure that grades out to a C+.

I pulled back my hand and slipped out of her embrace.

"This isn't right," I said.

She started to laugh. "You said it was *your* bungalow."

"It *is* my bungalow. But this isn't right."

"*Pffft.*"

"What?"

"You heard me."

"I don't know what you mean by it."

"I think it speaks for itself," she said.

I rolled my eyes. "Whatever you say."

She slapped me hard across the face.

I jumped up from the bed. "Why'd you do that?"

"You know why I did that," she said.

"No, Candy, I really and truly don't."

"But it's *your* bungalow. You said so yourself."

"Why don't I walk you back to *your* bungalow?"

She stood up. "I don't have a bungalow. My parents do."

"Then why don't I walk you back to *their* bungalow?"

"I know the way on my own."

With that, she stepped around me and walked out.

After she left, I sat in the twilight on the porch and tried to make sense out of what had happened. To no avail. The more I thought about it, the less sense it made. Then I caught sight of Perry making his way down the hill. He saw me sitting on the porch and hesitated. He held out both hands, palms upward; he was asking if it was safe to come inside.

I waved him forward.

"Did you get laid?" he said.

"Second base."

"That's good! That's good!"

"How did you know she was here?" I said.

"Robbie saw you walking with her."

"You'd think he'd have better things to do."

Perry sat down across from me and leaned back. He was smiling as though I were his prize pupil. Which, in a sense, I was. "So you got to second base with *Candy*. I never thought *anybody* would get that far with Candy. It's an accomplishment. Are you going to see her again?"

"Probably not," I said.

"Why? You got to second base. There's still a lot of summer left."

"It didn't feel right."

"It's your first tit," he said. "What do you have to compare with it?"

"No, the *situation* didn't feel right."

Perry rolled over the thought in his mind. Then at last he said, "If it doesn't feel right, it doesn't feel right."

"Well, it doesn't."

"But you got to second base. That counts for something."

He leaned forward and shook my hand. Then he stood up and walked back into the bungalow. Moments later, he returned to the porch with two cans of discount cola. We cracked them open, and, with great ceremony, Perry held up his can toward mine. "To Candy's tit."

I touched my soda can to his.

The news that I'd gotten to second base with Candy spread overnight among the camp staff and upended the common perception of me. The fact that I wanted nothing to do with her afterward led to the belief that I'd broken things off with her, rather than vice versa. Candy, for her part, did not care enough, or was too far gone, to correct that impression.

Whatever misgivings I might have felt over the entire incident soon evaporated. Girls were paying attention to me, if only to express their disapproval. One of Perry's first conquests, Miriam, sat down beside me during a snack break at camp and said, "I can't believe you'd do such a thing. *You!* I always thought you were sweet. But you took advantage."

It was the notion that they had misjudged me that finally put me on the radar of the teenage girls at Rosmarins; they'd taken me for an innocent, and I'd turned out to be a rogue. I experienced, for the first time, the pleasure of daily flirtations—a girl's hand tugging playfully at the side of my tee shirt, a girl's arm run casually around my waist, a girl's fingertips kneading the back of my neck. Each occasion caught me off guard. Each one, in retrospect, was pure bliss to dwell on. It struck me as a fair tradeoff: Sure, Perry had a half dozen notches on his bedpost, but there were complications. He had left a wake of hard feelings and heartaches, and I sensed remorse kicking in. I, on the other hand, had an ongoing stream of sexually charged moments to occupy my thoughts—as well as a relatively clear conscience.

I would have been content to wind down the summer under such circumstances except for a girl named Renee who entered the picture in late August. She had straight brown hair that fell almost to her waist, big brown guppy eyes, and a wide smile. She was startlingly thin, a wisp of a girl. I'd taken no notice of her because she was a counselor-in-training, a step below junior counselor, until she came up behind me late on a Friday afternoon. I was stacking Nok Hockey boards in the camp storage room, and she shoved her hands into the side pockets of my shorts. I startled at the sensation but did not move.

"I was just checking," she whispered in my ear.

"For what?"

"They said you had rubbers."

"What?"

"They said you always carry them."

"Who says that?"

"They do," she said, still whispering.

I turned to face her, which forced her hands out of my pockets. She was smiling up at me, knowingly.

"Well, I don't," I said.

She smiled. "I'm glad."

"Why?"

"I told them you weren't like that. I told them you were sweet."

"I'm glad I passed your test . . ."

"Renee."

"I'm glad I passed your test, Renee."

"Are you going to kiss me, or what?"

With a degree of trepidation, I leaned forward to kiss her. The next moment, her mouth was open, and mine was open in response, and a sudden heat was gathering in my lower abdomen unlike anything I'd felt before.

In a panic, I shook free of her.

"What are you doing?" I said.

"Don't you like being with me?"

"Yes."

"Don't you think I have a good body?"

"Yes."

"Can I see your bungalow?"

"Now?"

"Tomorrow night," she said.

"I suppose—"

"I'll be there at eight o'clock." She smiled mischievously, then ran her hand across my stomach and hurried out of the storage room. She left the door wide open, and a sudden wash of sunlight, like a curtain, appeared. I stared at the curtain of light, and the particulate dust it contained, and then at the open door. My heart pounded, but I did not move. Several moments later, I heard Perry's voice.

"Are you in there?"

"Yeah," I called.

He stepped into the storage room, passing through the light curtain, and looked at me in a strange way. "What happened to you?"

"Nothing."

"Must've been a lot of nothing," he said.

"Do you know Renee?"

"The C.I.T.?"

"Yeah, her."

"She wants to come down to the bungalow tomorrow night."

He narrowed his eyes. "She's a *C.I.T.*"

"What difference does that make?"

He began to sing, "*A younger girl keep rollin' 'cross my mind . . .*"

"C'mon, she's *one* year younger—"

"You don't know that she's fifteen. She could be fourteen."

"She's *not* fourteen," I said.

"How do you know?"

"Trust me, she's not fourteen."

"*No matter how much I try, I can't seem to leave her memory behind . . .*"

"It's not funny," I said.

"You've hit two bingos this summer. I'm just not sure about this one."

"Have I criticized your bingos?"

"Have you wanted to?"

"No, but I wouldn't even if I did."

"I'm not telling you what to do. I'm just telling you I'm not so sure."

Despite his reservations, Perry cleared out of the bungalow at seven thirty the next night—a half hour before Renee was due to arrive. He shot me a final look as he left, a lingering look that reiterated his doubts. It unsettled me. Perry's instincts had been dead on the entire summer; going against them now seemed stupid. But even if I wanted to back out, how could I? I had no clue where she lived. There wasn't enough time to ask around . . . and even if I lucked out and found the right bungalow in the first five minutes, I envisioned her father answering the door and inviting me inside for a chat. The prospect was unbearable.

So I sat on the porch and waited for Renee. I told myself that nothing was going to happen that I didn't want to happen; I tried to convince myself that that was the truth. But as eight o'clock drew near, I felt more and more like an actor in a play; I had lines to speak but no control over the outcome.

She came down the hill at one minute before eight o'clock. It wasn't quite dark outside but gray and shadowy. She wore a black tube top and short shorts, both of which accentuated her lack of curves. She *could* be fourteen, I thought. But did that matter? It was only a number. What difference did it make whether she turned fifteen after Labor Day or before Memorial Day? If what I was doing was wrong, it was wrong—regardless of the month she happened to be born. On the other hand, if it wasn't wrong, then it wasn't wrong.

Such was the state of my moral reasoning as she walked through the front door. I stood up and expected her to launch herself at me, but she hung back coyly, tracing her lower lip with her right index finger.

"You look sad," she said, instead of "hello."

"I'm not sad."

"I know how to make you happy."

"But I'm not sad."

"It's hot outside. My belly is sweating."

"Why do you think I'm sad?" I asked.

"Do you want to kiss my belly?"

"Do you want me to kiss your belly?"

She laughed sarcastically. "Yes, please."

I knelt down in front of her and kissed her stomach. It seemed a pointless exercise, just a test to see whether I would do it, until the moment my lips touched her skin. She moaned and began running her fingers through my hair. I was *affecting* her, making her moan. I thought of the many moans Perry had elicited that summer, the many and varied amorous noises that had echoed through the bungalow. Here, at last, was a contribution of mine. If the walls could talk, now they'd have cause to remember me.

"That feels so good," she said.

I stood up and looked her in the eyes. "Why do you think I'm sad?"

She threw her arms around my shoulders and began to kiss me. The sensation did not affect me as it had the previous afternoon. Instead, I hovered above the moment. I wondered whether the movements of her tongue were rehearsed, whether there was a method to them. Her eyes were open, and when our eyes met, she looked cross-eyed. I felt a smile form behind her kiss, and then she closed her eyes. I closed mine for a second but then opened them again. Out of politeness, though, I slipped my arms around her waist. Her response was to jump into my arms and wrap her legs around my hips. She was lighter than I thought she would be. She was straining and wriggling in my hands, kissing me frenetically, and I was in effect a bystander—intrigued by what she was doing, curious what she would do next, but unmoved.

After a half minute of holding her, I began to tire. I knew there was a cushioned chair no more than six inches behind me, so I took a quarter step backward and felt the seat against the back of my knees. As I sat down, she repositioned herself on my lap, with her legs outside of mine. She did not relinquish the kiss, however; she gave herself to it even more. Her abandon, in turn, further distanced me from the act. There were changes in her, of which I took note. Her breaths were more rapid. Her nostrils were flaring. Perspiration seeped from her face. From her forehead. From her cheeks. From her chin. Her moans were evolving into deep guttural growls. Abruptly, she stopped kissing me and pressed her mouth against my left shoulder. I could feel her teeth through the cotton of my tee shirt. For several seconds, she let loose a sound that was not quite a moan and not quite a sigh. I felt her tears, an instant later, through the cotton.

"Are you all right?" I asked.

Tears were rolling down both her cheeks, and she was laughing softly. "Yeah."

"That's as far as I want to go."

"What?" she said, as the focus returned to her eyes.

"I think we should go slow."

"What are you talking about?"

"There's no need to rush things."

"Don't you know what just happened?"

"We made out," I said.

She smiled and shook her head.

"All right, what happened?"

She kissed me on the forehead. "You're sweet."

She climbed off my lap and walked further into the bungalow. Moments later, I heard the bathroom door slide shut. That was followed by the sound of water rushing into the sink, and then the sound of the toilet flushing. I sat on the chair and listened, perplexed by what she'd said. Mostly, though, I felt relief. I had exercised my will, had made myself clear: We were *not* going to have sex that night.

Renee emerged from the bathroom and interrupted my reveries. She walked back out to the porch and pulled up a chair across from me. After a few seconds, she tilted her head to the side and said, "Penny for your thoughts?"

"I was thinking it's a warm night."

"What a gyp!"

"Sorry, I couldn't think of anything."

"Don't you want to get to know me?"

I rubbed the back of my neck with my right hand, then said, "You're not fourteen, are you?"

"I will be."

"What?"

"I'll be fourteen in October."

"You're *thirteen*?"

"Don't say it like that," she said.

"You're thirteen."

"I'm very mature."

"Yeah, but you're *thirteen*."

"You're still saying it like that."

"I'm *sixteen*."

"Well, you don't even know what just happened. So who's the immature one?"

"What are you talking about?"

"I think you're pretty lame for a sixteen-year-old if you don't know what just happened. I mean, you're supposed to have *experience*. I don't think we should go out anymore."

"We're not going out."

She stood up angrily. "I wouldn't waste my time!"

With that, she stormed out of the bungalow, slamming the screen door behind her.

For the next half hour, I replayed those five minutes with Renee—from the moment she walked into the bungalow to the moment she stormed out—sorting through the details while they were still fresh in my mind, trying to figure out what I'd missed, why she'd reacted the way she did, what had set her off. The one possibility that occurred to me was that she thought we'd had sex. She *was*, after all, only thirteen years old. But that explanation seemed too far-fetched. We'd made out; that was it. I hadn't gotten to second base, let alone third. For God's sake, we hadn't even taken off our clothes!

Could she be *that* naïve?

That was as far as I had gotten in my analysis when Perry came strolling down the hill. I heard his footsteps before I saw his outline underneath the darkness. I was torn about what to tell him. On the one hand, I was certain he'd have some critical insight into the situation; on the other hand, it seemed shameful to have made out with a thirteen-year-old.

He pulled open the door and said, "How did I know you'd wind up sitting on the porch, staring into space?"

"She only stayed five minutes," I said.

"What happened?"

"She was too young."

"Fourteen?"

"Not even," I said.

"Eek!"

"We kissed for a minute or so; that was it."

He rolled over the idea in his mind. "Well, that's not *too* bad."

"All we did was kiss."

"Tongue?"

I lowered my eyes. "Yeah."

"Did you hurt her feelings?"

"I don't think so," I said.

"You don't think she got attached?"

"No."

"'Cause thirteen-year-old girls get attached."

"She thinks she broke up with me," I said.

"Good! Good! How did you manage that?"

I shook my head. "I guess I lucked out."

Had the summer continued for another month, rather than for another week, word that I'd tongue-kissed a thirteen-year-old would likely have dissolved the reputation I'd acquired since my brief interlude with Candy. Renee did blab to whoever would listen, of course; she left out the specifics and just said that she'd gone to the bungalow, and that she and I had "fooled around." That was the phrase I heard whispered, and it resolved nothing. With Labor Day around the corner, in any event, no one cared much. What happened with Renee seemed a pardonable lapse in judgment—you do things you're not proud of as the summer is about to end.

The summer ended for Perry and me the Sunday before Labor Day. We spent the morning scrubbing clean the bungalow and packing our stuff into old suitcases and duffel bags. Except for a dollar bet on whose parents would arrive first—he bet on mine, and I bet on his—neither of us said a lot. The Rolling Stones filled the silences. Perry had ritually played the album *Exile on Main St.* from start to finish once every weekend the entire summer; he told me it would be good for my soul . . . yet another way he turned out to be right.

As the final notes of "Soul Survivor" sounded, he and I sat down on the porch and drank our last two discount colas. I was at a loss for words; I wanted to tell him that after a summer of thinking about sex and talking about sex, the only *love* I felt was for him But that's not the kind of thing one sixteen-year-old boy tells another. He must've sensed what I was thinking, because he smiled at me and said, "There's never going to be another summer like this."

"C'mon, there are going to be better summers."

"You're wrong."

"Why not?" I asked.

"Because we'll be older," he said.

"But that's why they'll be better!"

He laughed knowingly but didn't argue the point.

My parents turned up first, so I had to cough up the dollar. Perry helped me carry my suitcases and duffel bag out to the old Plymouth, which was parked at the top of the hill. I would've been content with a handshake, but he pulled me into a quick hug, punctuated by three pats on the back, then jogged back down the hill to await his parents. The last sight I had of him that summer was jogging down the hill toward our bungalow.

The drive back to Queens took a long time. We hit mile-long stretches of bumper-to-bumper traffic, turning the usual hour and a half into three hours. My mom and dad were bickering happily in the front seat; I sat in the back seat by myself, with the sun glinting intermittently into my eyes. What I was thinking was that they were bringing home a different guy than the guy they'd driven up to Rosmarins in June. Given what I'd experienced that summer, did it even make sense to still call them "Mom" and "Dad"? Weren't "Leona" and "Morris" more appropriate now? I mean, I was a man of the world. Within the next twelve months, I'd be driving by myself, graduating from high school, and starting college . . .

Maybe even figuring out what the hell had happened with Renee.

PUNCHING IN

Certain rhythms stick with you for your entire life. The tumbling trochees of "The Raven." The whir and crunch of a Slinky going down a staircase. The thumping bass line of Foghat's version of "I Just Want to Make Love to You." I picked up two unforgettable rhythms in June 1975:

Shove in, step down, let up, pull out
Whoosht-kih, whoosht-kih, whoosh-kih
Shove in, step down, let up, pull out
Whoosht-kih, whoosht-kih, whoosht-kih

The first was the mantra I spoke to myself as I stood in front of a drill press, eight hours a day, five days a week, punching holes in reams of loose-leaf paper: first, shove the paper into the press next, step on the treadle to bring down the triple drill bit; then, let up on the treadle to release the bit; and last, pull the paper out of the machine. The second rhythm was the relentless shift and clack of heavy machinery that surrounded me on the production line.

It was the first full-time job I ever held. The week after my freshman year of college ended, my father, in an act of Oedipal revenge, asked Yitzi, his nominal boss at Olympic Printing and Office Supplies, to hire me for the summer. The two of them hated each other—bosses and salesmen tend not to get along, because salesmen want to do things their own way, on their own schedule, and my dad in particular resented even the slightest whiff of supervision. But in this case their interests converged. Yitzi wanted minimum-wage labor, even if it was only for a couple of months. My dad wanted to teach me what hard work, what *real* work, felt like. So fresh off a spring semester in which I'd read Dostoevsky's *Notes from the Underground*, I found myself operating a three-hole drill press in an unventilated basement in Lower Manhattan.

To my left on the production line stood Jimmy G, who operated the main paper cutter. He was a middle-aged Sicilian with a five o'clock shadow that checked in by the morning coffee break, and with the darting eyes and twitchy muscularity of a mongoose. His was by far the most dangerous job on the floor. With both of his hands, he had to position stack after stack of finished broadsheets below a guillotine-length blade while he held down the blade's stopper with only his left foot. His foot had slipped off the stopper several times in the twenty-five years he'd worked the machine; only once had it cost him . . . the tip of his left pinky. It was a source of pride. He said guys who did his job had usually lost at least a couple of fingers, but he could still whack off the way God intended. Still, he didn't tempt fate. He made sure I knew, from the first day I joined the production line, what to do with a severed finger (pack it in ice; give it to the paramedics) if the situation arose.

To my right was Duncan. He was a huge black guy who hoisted, counted, and evened out the paper I'd just hole-punched and then fed the reams one by one into a machine that wrapped them in cellophane. He wore tee shirts with cut-off sleeves; the veins in his forearms pulsed visibly when he exerted himself. I estimated that he was in his late twenties, a number he'd neither confirm nor deny. He was good-natured about it, and I had the sense that he liked me, but he flat-out did not trust white people. He once told me that the best way to remember his name was to think about a yo-yo . . . and then to remember how the black man had been jerked around by the white man for the last three hundred years. Above his work station, he had an AM radio that blared soul music, and I will forever associate that job with three songs: "Fire" by the Ohio Players, "Low Rider" by War, and "Shining Star" by Earth, Wind and Fire.

The assistant foreman was Jose. He was in his forties with curly black hair and a wispy mustache. He was kindhearted and tolerant, but he spoke a language that was less a formal system than a blather of English verbs and Spanish nouns stirred into a syntax of his own devising. It left even the Puerto Rican delivery guys shaking their heads. Jose's language was both a handicap and an advantage. On the one hand, he often had to point and gesture to get you to do what needed to be done; on the other hand, he never had to justify what he was asking you to do. "Hey, Primo!" he would call, over the din of the machines. That meant I had to drop whatever I was doing and move one of the dozen cockroach-infested burlap garbage sacks out back to the loading dock for pickup at five o'clock. It made no sense; I was the weakest guy on the floor, by far, so I took twice as long to drag and shove the sacks to the dock. Still, the newest guy got the dirtiest jobs. That much I could respect, even if I could still feel imaginary roaches scampering up and down my arms for hours afterward. But pulling me away from my station caused the entire production line to grind to an abrupt halt. "Hey, Primo!" became the Spanglish equivalent of "Okay, let's take five!" Duncan would call it out to let Jose know he wanted a break, and Jose was often inclined to go along. He'd point me toward a half-full garbage sack, and that was that.

Jose's supervisor was Dominick, the production foreman. Dominick had a dingy metal office, more like an animal cage than a proper room, next to the loading dock. He came out only if there was a significant problem. The desire to keep Dominick in his cage was a great motivator among the dozen workers on the floor. He was the angriest man I'd ever met. His eyebrows were as thick as hedgerows, which, in their angles and arches, lent his rage a kind of vegetable substance; it was a *thing*, a force of nature that played across his face but seemed to originate elsewhere. He was in his late forties, had a boxer's nose, full lips, and pink splotches on his neck. He was not tall, no more than five feet, six inches, but he moved with the forward lurch of a tank and radiated physical power.

Dominick had a peculiar knack for keeping the machines working. He didn't fix them, exactly. But whenever one of the presses or cutters or feeders began to sputter or grind or jam, he would approach it with his hand on his chin. Calmly at first, he would size it up. He would listen to its noises. Walk a few circles around it. Turn a couple of knobs. He would switch it off and back on several times. Then, if the problem persisted, the rage would gather. It began with a swift kick at the base. Nothing premeditated. Just an exasperated tap with the toe of his shoe. Just hard enough to sting his foot. That would start the curses. Directed at the machine at first, and then directed at the universe in which he and the machine had been brought together, the curses soon became a torrent. That was the point at which the rest of us would stop what we were doing to watch—because we knew violence was at hand. He would lower his shoulder and ram the machine; it was bolted to the floor, of course, but Dominick, at five feet, six inches, was two hundred pounds of muscle, and the impact would rattle both of their insides. That would elicit more curses. He would spit into the gears of the machine, or hit the side with a forearm shiver, or drive his elbow into the control box. By then, Jose would have fetched his toolbox—which upped the ante. Dominick wouldn't use the tools except as weapons to continue his assault. He would bang and scrape and jab at the machine's innards. There was no logic to it. More often than not, however, the machine would start to work again. Suddenly, miraculously, the gears would mesh. The machine would come back to life. The bad noise would be gone. Dominick would step back and shake his head. For an instant, a look of affection would flash across his face. It was a good old machine, after all. He'd turn to whoever was operating it and mutter, "Keep her oiled from now on." Then he would retreat to his cage.

The list of things that ticked off Dominick, apart from broken machines, was long. The Yankees. The Knicks. The Giants. The Rangers. Shipment deadlines. Late deliveries. His paycheck. His wife. His unemployed son. His eighteen-year-old daughter—whom he'd warned me, the day I started the job, never to look at. But he took that back after the first month; he called me into his office late on a Friday afternoon, in a melancholy mood, and cursed the high school dropout she was dating. He said that if I wanted her number, he'd give it to me if I promised to treat her right. I made him that promise but declined the number. He nodded at me in an avuncular way. "You're not a scumbag," he said. "Don't let anyone ever tell you different."

What most got under Dominick's skin, on a day-to-day basis, was the collective he called "the Suits"—the supervisors and salesmen who worked upstairs. The fact that one of the Suits happened to be my father made no difference to Dominick. He told me what his opinion was; if his opinion upset me, or if I reported him, that just proved I was one of them. He didn't give a rat's ass what the Suits thought of him, he said. Even if I ratted him out, what were they going to do about it? Not one of them was man enough to look him in the eye and fire him. The Suits were nothing but pussies . . . though, paradoxically, they were also dicks and dickheads and motherfuckers.

Shove in, step down, let up, pull out
Whoosht-kih, whoosht-kih, whoosh-kih
Shove in, step down, let up, pull out
Whoosht-kih, whoosht-kih, whoosht-kih

I'd been on the job for six weeks when Dominick flung open the door to his cage for no apparent reason on a Friday afternoon. The door crashed into the side wall of the office, and the sound alerted us that he was on the floor. I did what everyone else did; I stared down at my machine and pretended not to notice. But I could hear his footsteps drawing near.

"Hey, kid!" he called.

I glanced up. "Me?"

"I'm borrowing you for a few minutes."

By then, he had walked past me, and I stood and watched him. I wasn't certain he wanted me to follow him; I didn't know if the few minutes had started, or if they were going to start at a time to be determined. So I waited to see if he would stop and turn around.

Several seconds later, he stopped and turned around. "You expecting an engraved invitation?"

"No," I said, switching off my machine.

I heard Jimmy G and Duncan laughing as I trotted after Dominick.

He was walking again as I caught up to him. "What's up?"

"They got a mouse upstairs," he huffed.

"A mouse?"

"Can you believe that shit? They got a fucking mouse, and they're calling me."

"Is it alive?"

"Right now, yeah," he said. "What a bunch of pussies!"

"You're sure it's not a rat?"

"I mean, am I their private exterminator? Call fucking pest control!"

As we were turning the corner to the stairwell that led to the sales floor, Dominick paused and reached behind him. I almost walked up his back. From the shadowed space beneath the first few steps, he pulled out a crowbar.

"What's that for?" I said.

"I'm going to pick my nose with it," he said. "What do you think it's for?"

"C'mon, Dominick."

"They want me to kill their mouse, I'm going to kill their mouse—my way."

"You can't kill a mouse with a crowbar—"

"Then I'm going to give it a bad fucking headache."

"C'mon, even if you do, you'll splatter it all over."

"You afraid of getting your socks wet?"

"Dominick, it's not sane."

He turned to face me, his eyes blazing. "Who the *hell* are you?"

Then he turned back around and marched up the stairs, the crowbar dangling at his side. I followed several steps behind him, shaking my head. Moments later, the two of us emerged into the piercing fluorescent light of the sales floor.

The entrance corridor was packed with more than a dozen employees—salesmen, secretaries, the two receptionists whose names I could never remember, the bookkeeper whose name I never knew, and Yitzi, who'd hired me. I was grateful not to find my dad among them; he'd cut out of work at three thirty to go to the racetrack, which was his habit on Fridays. They were chattering away when we appeared, the group of them, forcing jokes about the little mouse that had driven them from their desks. But they were spooked. That much was clear.

Yitzi stepped forward to meet us. Dominick's demeanor changed at once. He put out his hand, and Yitzi clasped it. "Hey, what do you know?"

"Sorry to bring you up here, Dom. I know this isn't your job—"

"Don't worry about it. I don't mind pitching in however I can."

Then Yitzi leaned forward and whispered something in Dominick's ear. I couldn't quite hear what he'd said, but it caused Dominick to smile and slap him on the back. That was also the moment when Yitzi caught sight of the crowbar at Dominick's side. He eyed the thing nervously. "You're not going to—"

"Nah, I might need to move a desk or two. They're bolted to the floor."

"Whatever you need to do," Yitzi said, with considerable relief.

"Where's the son of a bitch?"

"Toward the back. But he's been running all over . . . running wild."

Dominick grinned. "Then we'll have to put a stop to that."

Yitzi moved aside, and the two of us passed through the crowded corridor. I could feel the Suits inhaling to avoid contact with our bodies. Moments later, we stepped out onto the deserted main floor. The degree of difficulty became clear at once. The entire floor, except for the center aisle, was covered with brown carpet. There were six enclosed offices toward the back and another fourteen work stations set up along the center aisle. Each work station consisted of a metal desk surrounded on three sides by metal walls; these weren't cubicles, not in the prefabricated sense, but the intent was to divide the floor into private spaces. The worst of it, from our perspective, was that each dividing wall sat on rubber pads an inch above the floor . . . just high enough for a mouse to squirt underneath.

The mouse was going to be at a considerable advantage.

"Pussies," I heard Dominick mutter, once we were out of earshot of the rest.

"I don't think we're going to be able to find the thing—"

Before I could finish the sentence, however, the mouse darted across the bare floor of the center aisle and into the third work station on the left. The moment it hit the carpet, it seemed to dissolve into the brown pile.

Dominick strode in the direction of the mouse, grasping the crowbar with his right hand and slapping it into the meat of his left hand.

"What do you want me to do?"

"Find me a box!"

"What kind of box?"

"Big enough to hold a dead mouse."

After a quick scan of the floor, I noticed a cardboard shoebox beside the desk of one of the work stations. I hustled over to it; the box contained a pair of black high heels. I dumped the high heels onto the floor, snatched up the box, and rushed out to bring it to Dominick.

Just then, I heard the first dull thud of crowbar against carpet. It was followed by a second and a third.

"Fuck!" Dominick cried.

"Did you get it?"

Dominick came out of the third work station shaking his head in disgust. "Did it sound like I got it?"

"Where did it go?"

He nodded toward the back of the floor. "Somewhere down there."

The hunt was on . . . for Dominick at least. I held the shoebox under my arm and waited at the front of the floor, where the center aisle began; I was filled with a mixture of dread and fascination as he lumbered in and out of work stations, swinging the crowbar. There were more thuds and occasional crashes as he knocked over chairs and careened into sidewalls to cut down the angle on the mouse. Once, there was a loud clang, like the sound of a railroad tie being driven home, as he swung and caught only the bare floor of the center aisle; the crowbar went flying, and he let loose a wave of curses while he shook the sting from his right hand.

Now and then I'd catch a glimpse of the mouse scooting across the aisle, scurrying from work station to work station. On one occasion, it came tantalizingly close—maybe ten feet from where I stood. It occurred to me to drop the shoebox on it. But I knew Dominick would be furious if I took the mouse alive. The point was to splatter the thing. To splatter it and afterward hand the box to Yitzi. To shove the carcass in Yitzi's face, in front of his employees. That much had become clear.

What had also become clear was the unlikelihood that Dominick would ever get near the thing. I'd seen enough cartoons to know that Wile E. Coyote never splatters the Road Runner. That's not how the world works.

My reveries were suddenly interrupted by a hand that came down on my shoulder and spun me around. It was Yitzi. His eyes were livid, but he spoke to me in a whisper. "What the hell is that idiot doing?"

These were the first words he'd spoken to me since he hired me.

"Trying to kill the mouse," I answered, flatly.

"With a fucking crowbar?"

"I guess so."

"You're not too bright, are you?"

I shrugged my shoulders at him.

"Hey, Dom!" he called past me.

"Not now, Yitz!" Dominick called back.

"But you can't—"

"I'm *working* here! *Not now!*"

I'd never seen a face filled with more disdain than Yitzi's at that moment, but he said nothing else. He retreated to the entrance corridor with the rest of the Suits, and he left Dominick to his mayhem.

For the next several minutes, I continued to stand with the shoebox tucked under my arm and watched the scene unfold. The mouse scurrying from work station to work station. Dominick hustling after it, waving the crowbar and cursing in staccato outbursts. The overhead fluorescent lights bathed the entire floor in a surreal white glow, and I began to feel within me a profound indifference—a visceral indifference, if that's not a contradiction—to the outcome. The mouse's very existence was on the line. Dominick's pride, Yitzi's authority, these hung in the balance too. The stakes were high. Just not for me. Whatever happened, none of it had the slightest connection to me. After the summer, I'd be gone. Whether the mouse lived or died, whether Dominick and Yitzi resolved their power struggle, whether Jose learned English, whether Jimmy G kept his fingers, whether Duncan ever changed that radio station—the totality of it was irrelevant to the rest of my life.

But if *that* were true, I realized with a shudder, then the reverse also had to be true. My life meant nothing to them. The fact that I'd run track in high school. The fact that I'd never had sex. The fact that I'd read Dostoevsky. The epic saga that I seemed to be living, the long journey from innocence to experience, was passing unnoticed. Once the summer was over, once I was no longer in their midst, neither Dominick nor Yitzi nor Duncan nor Jose nor Jimmy G would give another thought to the outcome of my life. Perhaps no man is an island. But, with apologies to Donne, *every* man is a stream, a first-person narrative into which other narratives flow for a minute, or an hour, or a summer, or the greater part of a lifetime. It is at the intermingling of the waters that you define yourself: That story isn't mine. Here's my story . . .

For the first time, *Notes from the Underground* began to make sense. Life prepositions you in odd ways. No matter how logical your decisions, you still might wind up as the guy with a shoebox watching another guy with a crowbar chasing a mouse through an office. But here's the point. You aren't the sum of your prepositions. Ultimately, you are who you are.

The mouse darted across the aisle at that instant, and I lunged forward and flung the box at him. I missed, but Dominick saw me do it and rushed up to me. "What the hell was that?"

"I thought I had a chance."

"Nobody pays you to think."

"I did it anyway."

He stared at me; he hadn't expected an answer.

"You stay the fuck out of this."

I looked him dead in the eye. "You're never going to get that mouse, Dominick."

He wanted to curse me out, but he was out of breath. It gave him time to reflect on what I'd said. "You think you can do better?"

"Not with a crowbar, no."

"You think you can get the son of a bitch with that box?"

"Maybe," I said, "if you chase the son of a bitch toward me with the crowbar."

Despite himself, Dominick began to smile. "All right, we'll give your way a shot."

Instead of going after the mouse this time, he positioned himself one work station to the rear. I dropped to my knees with the shoebox in front of my chest. Then Dominick banged on the metal dividing wall with the crowbar. The mouse reacted, scurrying back across the center aisle. I lunged with the box and missed again, but only by a few inches. So we tried again, and again I missed. Dominick laughed out loud at my effort this time. "You're never going to play shortstop. I can tell you that for sure." He banged on the dividing wall again, and, again, the mouse bolted, and I lunged with the box . . . and caught the mouse.

"Got it," I called, matter-of-factly.

"You did not! You son of a bitch!"

Dominick wanted to take another swing at the mouse with the crowbar—through the shoebox—but I talked him out of it; I was the one who'd caught the mouse, so it was my call. He headed down to the production floor for rat poison. While he was gone, it crossed my mind to take the mouse outside and set it free. But I knew if I lifted the box, the mouse would get away, and we'd be back to square one. So I waited until he returned, and then I punched a hole in the shoebox with a fountain pen, and then he poured in the rat poison. For several seconds, I felt the mouse ricochet back and forth. Then there was quiet. Moments later, I lifted the box, and the mouse was dead.

Dominick sat down on the floor beside me. He said in a soft voice, "You have to give credit to the son of a bitch."

I laughed. "In what way?"

"He cleared out an entire floor of Suits."

"Yeah, he did."

"Plus, he sure outsmarted me."

"For a while," I said.

He clasped my left shoulder. "So I guess college teaches you something after all."

I smiled back at him. "I guess."

MANHOOD, PART THREE

The first time I ever fell in love, I skipped town. Twenty-two and as gullible as Elmer Fudd, I listened to nine months of promises that she would leave the fireman with whom she was cohabiting—until at last the truth began to dawn on me that girls don't leave guys who run into burning buildings for guys who work in bookstores and write unpublished novels.

So I went on a walkabout. Of course, I didn't know it was called a "walkabout"; *Crocodile Dundee*, the movie that popularized the term, didn't come out until 1986, six years later. But I knew, for the sake of my sanity and gastrointestinal well-being, I needed to get out of New York and see new stuff, so I scraped together several hundred dollars—a good chunk of my savings—bought a one-month unlimited-ride bus ticket at the Port Authority Bus Terminal in Manhattan, then hopped a Greyhound for points west.

My ultimate destination was Santa Barbara, California. I had a childhood friend there named Clyde Strong. He wasn't Clyde Strong when we were best friends on Thirty-Fourth Avenue; his name back then was a bit more, shall we say, circumcised. But he had left Flushing just after his high school graduation for Tampa, Florida, had done unsavory things there, the kind of things only guys like Clyde Strong get away with, and thus, by the time he re-settled in Santa Barbara, he'd gotten away with them and become Clyde Strong

There was another reason I wanted to visit Clyde, whom I hadn't seen in the flesh in over five years. He and I were barely out of diapers when we met and were inseparable for years afterward, but our friendship had waned during high school—he was the main supplier of hallucinogens for the block, and my abstinence antagonized him. In a moment of mutual sentimentality, he'd made me swear that if I ever smoked a joint I would do it with him, and I'd agreed.

I made that vow without knowing he would light out for the Territory. After he did, it slowly began to dawn on me that I was boxed in. Now, even if I *wanted* to smoke a joint, I was bound, in a *Horton Hatches the Egg* kind of way, to wait until Clyde was there to spark me up.

So I climbed aboard a Greyhound bus on the West Side of Manhattan bound for Santa Barbara, California. Up until that moment, the longest bus trip I'd ever taken was a three-hour charter from Queens College to Albany to protest proposed tuition hikes . . and that trip had just sailed by. I was with friends, and we played gin rummy, and after what felt like a half dozen hands, *voilà,* we were in Albany. (What happened in Albany, you ask? Well, we chanted and marched, but then the weather turned, and snow began to fall, and we got cold, so a couple of the organizers tried to set fire to a brass statue in front of the state capitol; when that fizzled out, we trudged back to the parking lot for the ride back to the city. I remember the Albany police pointing at us and laughing as the buses pulled out of the parking lot. Oh, and our tuition got hiked anyway.)

As I settled into a cramped seat near the back of the Greyhound bus for the ride to Santa Barbara, here's the gist of what I was thinking: *Three hours or three days, what's the difference? A bus ride is a bus ride.*

Plus, I had a deck of cards.

I'd play a half dozen hands, blink my eyes, and I'd be there . . .

The trip wasn't routed as the crow flies. It began with a seven-hour jaunt northwest to Cleveland, followed by a three-hour layover, followed by a twenty-three-hour butt-crippling meander southwest through Ohio, Kentucky, Tennessee, and Arkansas to Dallas, followed by another three-hour layover, followed by a *westward ho* death march across Texas, and then on to New Mexico, Arizona, and at last California and Santa Barbara.

Halfway across Pennsylvania, I tossed the deck of cards out the window. I hated the one-eyed jacks. *Personally*, I hated them. I suspected the girl who wouldn't leave her fireman boyfriend was fucking them. Why else were they winking at me?

So I decided to stare out the window, you know, to take in the grandeur of nature. The gentle, bosomy hills of central Pennsylvania. The lush, wind-combed meadows. The quaint farmhouses and silos. The cow pastures and even the occasional cluster of cows. Except here's the thing you realize coasting along at fifty-five miles per hour, staring out a bus window. Nature is indeed grand, but it's pretty damn repetitive. You walk down a single sidewalk in Manhattan, you see a hundred different things, with variations on variations. You roll down miles and miles of highway in Pennsylvania, you see about six things. Over and over and over. What I wouldn't have given for a glimpse of an Amish village, or a Hershey's factory. I'd have settled for Goober's Gas Station! But, no, it's just hills and meadows, farms and cows. Over and over and over.

So I turned inward. You can get a lot of thinking done riding alone on a bus. I had pretty much exhausted every thought I'd ever had, or ever would have, or ever cared to have, by the time the bus crossed from Pennsylvania into Ohio. Around Louisville, Kentucky, I scribbled this note to myself: "If water melts the Wicked Witch of the West, why doesn't she begin to dissolve from the moisture in Dorothy's hand the first time she grabs it?"

Around Nashville, Tennessee, I solved the riddle of what happens when an irresistible force meets an immovable object. It's a trick question: In a universe where an irresistible force can exist, you can't have an immovable object . . . and vice versa. *Ergo*, they can never meet. (I've since discovered that I wasn't the first person to come up with this solution.)

Around Little Rock, Arkansas, I gave up trying to stick my tongue in my navel.

Little Rock, however, provided a distraction because a young woman got on the bus. Midnight had come and gone as we pulled into the station, and the overhead lights flickered on, which caused me to roll down my sweatshirt. I noticed her as soon as I looked up. She was the only new passenger, and she stopped to talk to the driver as a half dozen other passengers exited through the rear door for bathroom breaks. While she and the driver chatted, I lost interest and closed my eyes. I didn't open them again until I heard the doors bang shut fifteen minutes later and felt the bus jerk forward. When I looked up, the young woman was headed toward me. She had a long brown duffel bag slung over her shoulder as she made her way down the aisle. I didn't want her to notice me noticing her, so I turned to face the window and watched her in reflection—one of the subtler horrors of riding a cross-country bus at night is the fact that the dim light inside is always brighter than the pitch black outside, so the windows become mirrors; you get to see yourself grow more and more haggard.

The bus wasn't crowded. Entire rows were empty, but the young woman walked past them. She stopped next to me, shoved the duffel bag into the overhead storage bin and sat down across the aisle. I continued to study her in reflection. She was roughly my age, with wide-set brown eyes, a cascade of dark brown hair, a gray shirt that bared a six-inch section of her midriff, and jeans. She went through a sequence of stretches, arching her back, twisting her shoulders, bringing her legs to her chest, rolling her head from side to side; the entire performance was too feline for words. Once she'd gotten comfortable, she began to eye me. This went on for several minutes.

Then, at last, she said, "You probably want to strike up a conversation, don't you?"

I turned around to face her. "What makes you say that?"

"Because you're not doing anything else."

"I guess I wouldn't mind a conversation."

"You don't ride the 'Hound much," she said.

"Not as much as I have lately."

"Where'd you get on?"

"New York City," I said.

"Wow!"

"Wow, that's a long way? Or wow, New York?"

"Both, I guess. You don't look like New York."

That made me laugh, which brought a twinge of pain; my facial expression hadn't shifted in hours, and the muscles had settled. She started to twist the ends of her hair into tighter curls.

"You're a college boy, right?"

"Not anymore," I said.

"Dropped out?"

"Something like that."

"Let me guess. You fell in love, and you dropped out, and then things didn't go like you planned, so you said 'to hell with it,' and you got on a bus. You don't even know where you're going, right?"

"Close enough," I said.

"I'm very empathic."

I put out my hand. "I'm Mark."

"Margie." She shook my hand.

"Where are you going?" I asked.

"I've got friends out West," she said. "I'm going to spend a couple of months with them."

"Are you in college?"

She cracked up. "That'll be the day! Nope, not going to happen. I didn't even stick around for my last year of high school. I'm more a classroom-of-life kind of gal, if you get my drift. How long do you want to talk for?"

"Until we run out of stuff to say."

"Sounds good to me," she said.

"Where out West do your friends—"

"I'm guessing you've had sex, what, ten times? Maybe twelve?"

"Huh?"

"You don't have a lot of sexual experience, am I right?"

"What makes you say that?"

"You're avoiding the question!"

"I'm not avoiding—"

"You don't have to answer it. I just thought you wanted to talk."

"I have no idea how many times I've had sex," I said.

Actually, I did . . . four.

"You seem like a guy who needs to have sex a few more times."

"In order to do what?"

"In order to not worry so much about sex," she said.

"You're the one who brought up the subject!"

"It was already out there. I told you . . . I'm very empathic."

"I don't even know what that word means—*empathic*. Is it the same thing as empathetic?"

"No, they're completely different words."

"What does *empathic* mean?"

"It means I *get* people," she said. "I feel what they feel."

"Isn't that what *empathetic* means?"

"Really? I thought they were completely different. I guess I'm both."

"Maybe you should join the circus."

"Look, I'm sorry if I hurt your feelings. I didn't intend it as a criticism. I thought it might be an interesting topic to talk about."

"You didn't hurt my feelings," I said.

She smiled at me. "You sure I didn't hurt them? Not even a little bit?"

Her smile got to me. "Maybe a little bit."

"You see?" She pointed at the side of her head. "Empathic."

We talked the entire five and a half hours from Little Rock to Dallas. I steered the conversation clear of my love life, and Margie turned out to be good company. She held unorthodox views on popular music (Lynyrd Skynyrd, not Elvis Presley or Bob Dylan or the Beatles, had been the defining act of the rock era), politics (elected officials should be forced to take a vow of celibacy for as long as they held office), and religion (Jesus had been an alien.. . . "Read Erich von Däniken, and then read the gospels. It makes perfect sense!"). She gestured broadly as she spoke, and whenever she said something that struck her as profound or irrefutable, she would lick her index finger and swipe it in the air, as if she'd just scored a point.

It was a few minutes past five in the morning, and we were a half hour from Dallas, when she looked straight at me and said, "So do you want to get off the bus?"

"Why?"

"We can split a hotel room," she said. "Take hot showers. Sleep in real beds."

"How much do you think that would cost?"

"Twenty-five apiece would likely cover it."

"Do you know a hotel in Dallas?"

"No, but we can ask at the station," she said. "There's always a hotel in walking distance from the bus station. If you've got a bus station, you've got a hotel in walking distance. It's the most obvious place to put a hotel."

"Do we have to pretend to be married?"

"C'mon, it's *1980*!"

"What does that mean?"

"It means I'm not Doris Day, and you're not Rock Hudson, and no one cares."

"Oh," I said . . . and meant it.

"Well?"

It occurred to me, of course, that splitting a hotel room might be a euphemism for having sex, especially following her diagnosis that I needed more of same. But I wasn't certain. She'd said that we would be able to sleep in "clean beds"—the plural seemed significant. There was the further complication that my heart still belonged to the girl who lived with the fireman . . .

"Count me in," I said.

The Hotel Lawrence was a block from the Dallas terminal, which seemed to confirm Margie's theory of hotels in proximity to bus stations. I waited at the far end of the deserted lobby—it was just after six in the morning—while she walked up to the front desk and booked us a room. Three minutes later, she came back proudly dangling a set of keys.

"I flirted with him, and he gave us a free ride for the rest of the morning," she said. "We don't have to check out until noon, tomorrow."

"How much was it?"

"Forty-five dollars. Can you cover thirty?"

"Yeah," I said.

"Thanks, I'm a little cash-strapped."

After a couple of wrong turns, we found the room at the end of a long hallway on the third floor. Margie opened the door, and I followed her inside. There was only one bed, queen size, in the center of the room. There was a couch, not quite long enough to sleep on, along the far wall near the window. Without acknowledging the awkwardness of the configuration, Margie flung her duffel bag onto the bed, and I dropped my backpack onto the couch.

Then she turned to me—we were dangerously close as she spun around—and said, "Mind if I hit the shower first?"

"Not at all," I answered.

She was turning back around and kicking off her shoes while the words were still hanging on in the air, to which I responded with a kind of showy indifference. *Nothing to see here. Just another pretty girl stripping off her clothes within my peripheral vision.* . . . I sat down on the couch and yawned. Then I began fishing through my backpack. I found my wallet at the bottom, took out my driver's license and slid it into a different compartment in my wallet. I had no reason for doing this. But it gave me the appearance of being busy. Afterward, I slid the wallet into my pants pocket.

"I don't mind if you look," she called.

"I know," I said. But I didn't look. I concentrated on a street lamp that loomed just below the window. It had an amber bulb and cast the ceiling of our room in a kind of jazz-club glow.

"It's just the human body. It's nothing to get uptight about."

I glanced back at her, but only for a second. She was down to her bra and panties.

"You're very pretty," I said.

She smiled. "You're sweet."

With that, she stepped into the bathroom and shut the door softly behind her. The shower came on a moment later, and only then did I shift my attention from outside to inside. There was an almost studied quality to the haphazard mess of her clothes. One pink sock was strewn across the floor; the other was hanging from the doorknob of the closet. Her jeans were folded neatly over the footboard of the bed, but her gray shirt was wadded up into a ball near the pillows. She had left her bra and panties in a pile at the threshold of the bathroom.

She took a *long* shower. For the first half hour, I sat on the couch and tried not to over-think the situation. I pulled the Gideon's Bible out of the nightstand and flipped through the gospel according to Matthew, trying to find hints of an extraterrestrial Jesus. Then my curiosity got the better of me, and I tiptoed over to the bathroom. I put my ear to the door and listened. The shower was still running full blast, but I could also hear her singing underneath the roar of the water. It took me a couple of seconds to recognize the song: "I Love the Nightlife." She was warbling, "Please don't talk about love tonight . . . please don't talk about *sweeeeeet* love . . ."

Maybe a minute later, the rush of water stopped, and I heard her step out of the shower. I hurtled back across the room to the couch, where I leaned back and pretended to be half asleep. It was another minute until the bathroom door opened, and a cloud of steam billowed into the room.

Wrapped in a long white towel, Margie emerged from the bathroom. She was barefoot, and her hair was a tangle of wet curls.

She smiled at me coyly and said, "Your turn."

I jumped off the couch and headed for the bathroom. As I passed her, I noticed a tiny black tattoo on her left shoulder.

"Is that a swastika?" I said.

"No, it's that German thing."

"You mean a swastika."

"Is that what it's called?"

"Yeah," I said. "But why—"

"All my friends were getting them a couple of years ago," she said. "It was like a group thing we did together."

"Do your friends ride motorcycles?"

"Most of them. How'd you know?"

"Just a hunch," I said.

"I guess it could be taken the wrong way—"

"I'm not sure there's a *right* way to take it."

"You're saying that 'cause you're from New York. You need to get out of the city more often."

I shrugged.

Yeah, I know, but what else was I going to do? Debate her on the peculiar evil of the Holocaust? At six thirty in the morning in the Hotel Lawrence in Dallas? While she was wrapped in a towel, and her hair was dripping onto the carpet? Besides, I just wanted to get into the bathroom. Not only did I want to shower, I *needed* to pee.

So I brushed past her and started to unbuckle my belt. I was planning a grand display of nonchalance . . . I was going to drop my jeans and pull off my sweatshirt at the threshold of the bathroom door, leave them in a rumpled pile, then step into the bathroom in my tighty-whities alone. Two could play at this *it's-just-the-human-body-nothing-to-get-uptight-about* game.

But as I was unzipping my fly, I paused. Right then, within the space of a moment, I formulated Goldblatt's Law: *Never take off your pants in a hotel room with a girl with a swastika tattoo.*

I stepped into the bathroom still clothed and locked the door behind me, then double-checked it. Feeling relatively secure, I turned on the water in the shower and got naked.

As soon as I stepped into the shower, I understood why Margie had taken so long to come out of the bathroom. The showerhead was equipped with a pulsating massage option, and the water pressure for the hotel must have been set at *thwart-a-civil-rights-protest*—I'd never been hit that way by a liquid. The sensation was stunning, quasi-religious. The rotating jets seemed to knead the contours of the bus seat from my back and to peel away the highway miles from my skin. When I turned my head from side to side, the pulses drove straight into my ears and pounded life back into my brain.

I was at least twenty minutes, and three latherings, into the shower when I heard the door of the hotel room slam. It took perhaps five seconds before the meaning of the sound registered . . .

I'd been robbed.

Now, at once, the entire interlude with Margie came clear. The reason she'd struck up the conversation on the bus. The reason she'd hinted at a sexual liaison. The reason she'd suggested getting off at Dallas. The reason she'd asked to shower first. The reason she'd made a show of stripping off her clothes. Ah, but I'd had the last laugh, because my jeans, with my wallet in the pocket, were lying on the floor of the bathroom, and the door was locked, and the contents of the backpack with which Margie had made off—three tee shirts, a pair of gym shorts, another pair of jeans, three changes of underwear and socks, a can of deodorant, a yellow notepad, and a couple of pens—would likely net her about ten dollars on the open market. Of course, I'd have to cover the full cost of the hotel room, and afterward I'd have to replace the backpack and its contents, which was going to set me back much more than ten dollars, but the lesson I'd learned was, in the greater scheme of things, worth the cost.

I realized all of that in the first half minute after I heard the door slam.

Then I thought about the swastika tattoo, and how, if I hadn't seen it, I would have left my jeans, and thus also my wallet, outside the bathroom door, and I realized that the swastika, and thus also, in a roundabout way, Hitler and the Nazis, had saved me.

Still, I didn't rush out of the shower. The water felt too warm against my skin, and besides, what was the point? Was I going to run dripping wet into the hotel lobby, yelling that I'd been robbed? *Yeah, that girl I checked in with an hour ago, at six o'clock in the morning, she robbed me. No, I don't know her last name. But you remember her, right? The pretty one, with the curly brown hair and the swastika tattoo. She made off with my gym shorts!*

So I sighed, and moved even closer to the showerhead, and let the water smack me around for another ten minutes. The upside, I was thinking, was that I had the hotel room to myself, that I'd be able to sleep on the queen-size bed rather than on the couch. I was also wryly amused at the fact that my life had become a country-and-western lyric: "I got rolled in the Hotel Lawrence/in the dawn of a Texas morning." (Though, of course, you'd have to drop the *g* in *morning.*)

Reluctantly, I stepped out of the shower. It took a minute to dry my hair with a hand towel, and then I cinched the last large white towel around my waist and stepped back out into the room.

Margie was lying on a metal cot, with the covers pulled up to her chest, off to the side of the queen-size bed. Her swastika tattoo was peeking out over the top sheet. She looked up at me and smiled. "I figured you deserved the real bed since you were paying most of the money."

"Where'd you get the cot?"

"I ordered it when we checked in. The guy said there was only one bed."

"What? But I thought . . ."

She smiled. "What did you think?"

"I thought . . . I don't know.. . . I heard the door slam . . ."

"I wouldn't call for room service without asking you."

I sat down on the edge of the bed, feeling as low as I'd ever felt. "When I heard the door slam, I thought . . ."

"C'mon, you can say it."

"I don't want to say it."

"You thought I'd stolen your stuff, right?"

"Yeah."

"Well, I definitely *could* have," she said. "If you look at the thing objectively, you were pretty naïve to trust me. On the other hand, you could've been a killer-rapist, so I guess we both kind of lucked out."

I shook my head and took a deep breath. "You sure you don't want the bed? I feel like I should take the cot."

"No, I'm already tucked in. But thank you for being such a gentleman. Oh, and thank you for not being a killer-rapist."

I pulled down the covers and slid into the bed, then dropped the bath towel onto the floor. "Good night."

"Good night, New York," she said.

Margie and I slept through the entire morning and well into the afternoon, then ate breakfast-dinner together, watched reruns on TV until three a.m., slept through the next night, and went our separate ways the following morning. We parted at the bus station, minutes before the bus was scheduled to leave. I'd thought we were getting back on the bus together, but she turned without warning and gave me a sudden, desperate hug. When she pulled back, her eyes were damp. "You take care of yourself, New York."

"You're not going to visit your friends?"

"They can wait," she said. "I'm going to stick around here for another few days."

"Why? What's here?"

"Just because . . . and that's what I want to figure out."

"Where are you going to stay?"

"I'll figure that out too," she said.

"Do you need money?"

"What did I tell you about being naïve?"

She kissed me lightly on the cheek, turned, and walked out of the bus terminal.

I never saw her again.

I boarded the Greyhound in Dallas at seven forty-five that morning and hunkered down for the rest of the trip to Santa Barbara, California. First, however, there was the little matter of getting out of Texas. Until you've ridden a bus across Texas, it's hard to grasp how big it is. It's hard to grasp how big *big* is. If you trace the bus route on a map, what you see is the graceful southwest swoop of Route 20—through Forth Worth, through Abilene, through Sweetwater, through Big Spring, through Odessa, and through Pecos. Going by the names alone, you keep expecting to pick up a cussing sidekick called Smiley or Gabby or Stumpy.

No such luck.

Riding across west Texas makes riding across Pennsylvania feel like the chariot race scene at the end of *Ben Hur*. West Texas is where *ad nauseum* meets *ad infinitum*. It's prairies and farms, followed by prairies and farms, followed by mileage markers and shrubs, followed by prairies and farms. You stare out the bus window, and nothing gets in the way of your view . . . of nothing. There's nothing there. Just miles and miles and miles of West Texas nothing.

Miles and miles and miles of gaze-hardening, brain-braising, soul-flattening, West Texas nothing. What was it like? Imagine being forced to read a three-hundred-page book of blank pages. You flip through the pages, one by one, just to make sure each page is blank, until you get to the end. Sounds like a pain in the butt, but you can get through it, right? Except imagine you have to spend several minutes on each page . . . and you have to get to the end of the book before your life can continue.

It's like that, but with recycled air and intermittent coughing.

The bus lurched and sputtered into the station at El Paso a mere twelve hours after we'd left Dallas. (That's just past sunrise to just past sunset, a half rotation of the earth, if you're keeping score at home.) I stepped off for a bathroom break and overheard a couple of guys who'd been sitting a row in front of me arguing about whether to hike over the footbridge to Juarez and get laid. The getting laid part seemed to be a given; what they were debating was whether the hour layover in El Paso gave them enough time to get back to the bus.

I was intrigued by this bridge to getting laid and thought it would be worth looking into, even though the prospect of crossing it filled me with ambivalence. I noticed the bus driver ordering a cup of coffee in the terminal and asked him where the bridge was. He said it was only a few blocks away, but he recommended against the hike because Juarez was dangerous, especially if you didn't know where you were going.

"I've seen guys get stabbed a minute after they set foot in Mexico," he said. "The locals pick out the easy marks."

That cinched it for me: I might have been ambivalent about getting laid, but a knife wound would break up the monotony of the rest of the ride to Santa Barbara, so off I went.

The price for crossing the footbridge from the United States to Mexico was five cents. You didn't need to show a passport or I.D. of any kind. You paid your nickel, and you took your walk. The bridge itself was about three football fields long, poorly lit, and scattered with clusters of young men; there was some joking back and forth among them, but most of the voices I heard were subdued—they sounded like I'd sound if I were on my way to Mexico to get laid.

I was on my way to Mexico to get stabbed, however so I was relaxed.

As I came to the last twenty-five feet, I could already hear catcalls from prostitutes on the Juarez side: "Want to fuck with me, *muchacho*?" and "I've got a sweet pussy for you!"

That was when I decided I didn't want to get stabbed badly enough to go through the hassle of explaining my situation to the locals, so I turned back. I never quite made it to Mexico.

Half an hour after the bus left El Paso, we crossed the New Mexico border, and the long sojourn through Texas was over. I fell asleep when I heard the bus driver make the announcement—comforted by the knowledge that Texas did indeed end—and slept the rest of the night. I fought off the glints of dawn as long as I could, until I was sure New Mexico and Arizona were in the rearview mirror. When, at last, I opened my eyes, we were in California.

The last leg of the trip—from Blythe, just across the California-Arizona border, to Santa Barbara, where Clyde Strong and my first joint awaited—was a blur. I experienced the peculiar sensation of leaning at the tape for nine hours. Still, I had daylight, and I had things to see out the window. Weather-worn billboards and sand dunes dotted with litter and fresh-fruit stands. Palm trees swaying in the breeze—just like the ones I'd seen on *Gilligan's Island*! Hell, there were even towns every dozen or so miles. After West Texas, it felt like sensory overload.

Then, at last, at four o'clock in the afternoon, we rolled into the Greyhound station in Santa Barbara. I climbed off the bus for the last time, dropped my backpack, knelt down, and kissed the sidewalk. It tasted like sidewalk. When I looked up, Clyde Strong was standing over me, smiling.

He lifted me to my feet and hugged me for a long time. I hugged him back and sobbed a couple of times. They were free-floaters, the sobs. I didn't know they were in me until they were out, and Clyde hugged me even harder when he heard them. "Why didn't you fly?" he said.

It was a fair question; I had no good answer. Counting the cost of the hotel room in Dallas, the breakfast-dinner I'd eaten with Margie, the prepackaged sandwiches and potato chips I'd bought along the way, and the nickel I'd paid to walk to Juarez, I'd spent the difference between an unlimited-ride bus pass and a round-trip plane ticket.

I looked Clyde in the eye and shrugged.

"C'mon," he said. "Let's go back to the house and get you washed up. You stink."

Clyde drove me back to his house in a maroon Cadillac convertible. It was the first time I'd ever ridden in a convertible, and after thousands of bus miles, I was grateful for every second of the wind in my face.

"Nice car," I said, as we exited the highway.

"It's used, but it gets me from here to there."

"I don't even know what you do for a living."

He glanced across the front seat. "I do a little bit of this and a little bit of that."

"Oh."

Clyde lived at the top of a steep hill in a long flat house with beige walls and a terra-cotta roof. He flicked a switch on his keychain as we started up the driveway, and the door to one of the two garages rolled up.

"What do you think?" he said.

"You *own* this place?"

"Owning is for suckers. I rent."

"Isn't it kind of . . . huge?"

"I've got roommates," he said.

"Oh."

He parked the car and motioned me through a side door in the garage that led into the house. We walked along a narrow corridor, past a stacked washer and dryer, and then past a long clothesline strewn with women's underwear. We emerged into the kitchen. There was a woman who looked disconcertingly like Adrienne Barbeau washing lettuce over the sink. She smiled as soon as she noticed us.

"Hey, boy! Who's your friend?"

Clyde walked up behind her and pressed himself into her backside. "He's not my friend, baby doll. He's my *best* friend, and his name is Mark, and don't you forget it. You hear me, Babs? Now, spell it for me."

"M-a-r-k, right? Or is it with a *c*?"

"With a *k*," I said.

"I'm pleased to meet you, Mark-with-a-*k*. Any *best* friend of Clyde's is a *best* friend of mine."

Still standing behind her, Clyde wrapped his arms around her and cupped her breasts through her tee shirt. She moaned loudly and turned her head enough to flick her tongue in his ear. She did not let go of the lettuce, however.

After several seconds, he unhanded her.

"Are you boys going to stick around for dinner?"

"Don't know," Clyde said.

"Well, if you want, there's plenty to go around."

"There's always plenty to go around with you!"

"C'mon, Clyde . . ."

"Bounce for me, Babs!"

Babs twisted her torso in my direction and gave her breasts a quick shake.

"What did I tell you, Mark?" Clyde shouted, happily.

He hadn't told me about Babs. I'd have remembered.

We left the kitchen and headed toward the rear of the house and a long hall lined with bedrooms. As I was about to ask Clyde about Babs, two more women stepped out of separate bedrooms and into the hall. The taller one was Nordic, a younger, ganglier facsimile of Inger Stevens, the sort of no-question-about-it-natural-blond who looks like she's perpetually about to go skiing. The shorter of the two was Hispanic . . . or Arab . . . or Asian; I kept changing my mind depending on the angle at which she turned her head.

They both smiled at Clyde the same way Babs had smiled at him.

"This is my best friend, Mark," Clyde said. "I want you to treat him right. Do you understand? He's my *best* friend in the entire world. We go back *forever*. He's knows all my secrets."

"*Ooh!*" they chorused.

"Well," I said, "I'm not sure I know *all* your secrets."

"We're going to grill you anyway," the shorter woman said. "I'm Halima."

The taller woman stepped forward and put out her hand. "Hello, I'm Beth."

I shook Beth's hand and reached for Halima's. But Clyde yanked me by the sleeve toward his bedroom, which was the last one at the end of the hall. I wound up waving at Halima.

"You live with three women?" I whispered.

"Five," he said. "But who's counting?"

"*Five?*"

"Or six. It depends on the day of the week."

He pushed open the door to his room and led me inside. There was a worn-out blue couch pitched against one wall, a wooden board that served as a desk resting on stacks of cinder blocks, and a tray table with a film projector in the middle of the room. That was it. There was nothing on the walls except cracks in the plaster.

"The couch folds out into a bed," Clyde said. "I put clean sheets on it, so you won't get my cooties. Except maybe I should be more worried about your cooties. You stink."

"Where are you going to sleep?"

He smiled at the question. "I'll figure something out."

"Is Babs your girlfriend?"

"Not right now," he said.

"But the way you—"

"You have to let go of labels, Mark. Labels are what make you crazy. They don't mean anything anyway. She's who she is, and I'm who I am, and whatever happens happens."

"What about Beth and Halima?"

"Same story, different verses."

"But how can that be?" I asked.

"It's just sport fucking," he said. "It's no big deal."

I didn't know how to respond to that, so I let it go.

"Thanks for putting me up," I said.

"Hey, you can move in if you want."

"My life is back in New York City."

"You mind if I ask you a question?"

"No," I said.

"You didn't *really* ride three thousand miles on a Greyhound bus to smoke a joint."

"That's not a question."

"Don't get me wrong," he said. "I'm glad you're here. But I wasn't going to hold you to that stupid promise."

I laughed. "You could've mentioned that over the phone."

"When a guy calls you up and tells you he's going three thousand miles out of his way to smoke a joint, you don't grill him about the real reason. You get out your rolling paper and tell him to come on down."

"I appreciate it," I said.

"So who ripped out your heart?"

"If I told you her name, would it matter?"

"No," he said.

"Then what's the point of my telling you?"

"Do you want me to get you laid?"

"That won't be necessary," I said.

"So it's just the joint, and then *sayonara*?"

"Well, I *do* have a bus to catch . . ."

He waved his hands. "Do what you got to do. I'm just saying if you want to get laid, I can make it happen."

"Let's focus on the shower first.. . . I stink."

"Third door on the right, or fourth door on the left. Knock first, because the girls don't believe in locks. Oh, and there's another bathroom downstairs in the basement just in case."

He snapped his feet to attention and gave me a mock salute, then turned and headed out the door.

As soon as he was gone, I pulled out a change of clothes from my backpack and found the third door on the right. I knocked twice, then called to whoever was in earshot that I was about to take a shower. I locked the door behind me, but I wasn't certain that the latch had caught. Still, the bathroom door was clearly shut, and I'd indicated in a loud voice what my intention was. For a moment, I considered taking a bath; the idea of soaking in a tub, after the last leg of the bus ride, was tempting. But it seemed rude to monopolize one of the bathrooms so soon after I'd arrived. I stripped down, played with the hot and cold faucets until the temperature felt right, and then stepped through the shower curtain and into the shower.

I'd been at it for maybe five minutes, with lather in my hair and running down my face, when I heard a hard knock at the door.

"I'm showering," I called out, tasting shampoo with each syllable.

"It's just me," came a woman's voice.

"Who's *me*?"

"Beth. You know. We just met."

"I'll be out in another five min—"

The door abruptly swung open; I felt the cold air from the hall sweep around the shower curtain. Reflexively, I jumped to the back corner of the tub, nearest the faucet, and dropped into a crouch, using both elbows to cover my groin.

"I just need to pee," Beth called to me.

"Um . . ." I gulped down a mouthful of lather, then coughed it up.

"Hey, are you all right back there?"

"Um . . . yeah."

"I'll just be a second," she said.

The shower curtain was a frosted gray, translucent but not transparent. Still crouched over, I rubbed the suds away from my eyes; I could make out the shape of Beth's body. She was perched on the toilet, going about her business. I couldn't hear her, but there was no question that she was in fact peeing. I had never seen a woman urinate. I began to feel guilty watching her, even with the shower curtain between us. She seemed to be paying no attention whatsoever to me.

Warily, I rose up out of the crouch, covering my groin with my hands instead of my elbows. I didn't quite resume showering, but I stepped under the water to give the appearance of showering. I also averted my eyes, staring up at the patch of white tiles just above the shower nozzle.

I heard the toilet flush, and I exhaled: *No big deal*, I thought.

But an instant later, Beth grabbed the edge of the shower curtain and yanked it open. This time, I spun around and dropped down into the tub in a seated position. I hunched over and pressed myself so close to the side that the stream of water was no longer getting me wet.

"What are you *doing*?" I yelled, looking up.

She was giggling. "Sorry, I just *had* to know."

"Know *what*?"

"If you were, you know, like Clyde."

"What are you talking about?"

She giggled again but didn't answer. Then she let go of the shower curtain, turned, and walked out of the bathroom.

I sat in the tub for at least three minutes, trying to figure out what had happened and waiting to see what would happen next. Then, keeping one eye on the door, I grabbed the soap out of the soap dish and hastily finished showering. I dried myself and got dressed as fast as I could, then darted from the bathroom back to Clyde's room. He was sitting on the couch, smiling at me.

"Beth said she checked you out," he said. "Sorry about that."

I shook my head. "Why would she do something like that?"

His smile got wider. "You'd have to ask her."

"Is she crazy?"

"Beth? Nope."

"You're not trying to get me laid, are you?"

"Nope."

I sat down on the couch next to him. "She said she wanted to know if I was like you. What does that mean?"

"You don't want to know."

"I *do* want to know," I said.

"Trust me, Mark, you don't."

His tone got under my skin. "What the hell are you doing here, living with five women? Are you Charles Manson?"

"It's nothing like that," he said.

"Then tell me what's going on."

"Look, why don't you ask Beth what she meant?"

"I will!"

"Well, you know where she lives."

I walked out of Clyde's room, headed up the hall and stopped at the door I was ninety-nine percent sure Beth had come out of. I was about to knock but hesitated. What if I *didn't* want to know the answer?

No, I definitely *did* want to know.

I knocked twice on the door.

I recognized Beth's voice on the other side. "Yes?"

"It's Mark . . . Clyde's friend . . ."

She pulled open the door. "I know who you are."

"Why did you do that in the bathroom?" I said.

"I told you. I had to pee."

"No, the other thing."

"You mean why did I sneak a peek?"

"Yeah, that," I said.

She looked at me in a sly way. "Come on in."

I followed her into the room. Unlike Clyde's room, Beth's looked like it had been given a moment's thought. The walls were decorated with framed movie posters, abstract art, and a full-length art deco mirror. There were several shelves of books, a dresser, a chest of drawers, and a rolltop desk. Beth sat down on the edge of the platform bed, and she patted the mattress beside her and motioned for me to sit next to her. Still feeling uneasy, I sat down.

"All right," I said. "I'm listening."

"Can I ask you a question first?"

"Go ahead."

"When you were a kid, what did you call a penis?"

"Is that a joke?"

"No, I want to know. What word did you use?"

"I used the word *penis*," I said.

"You didn't call it a dick, or a cock, or wiener?"

"No, I pretty much stuck with *penis*."

"So here's the thing," she said. "Your friend Clyde has the biggest penis I've ever seen."

"What?"

"It's *huge*!" She held out her hands a foot apart.

"C'mon . . . Clyde?"

"I swear. It made me cry the first time I saw it."

"*That's* why you—"

"I wanted to see if maybe you guys had a club or something."

"No, we didn't," I said.

"Well *that's* obvious."

It took a split second for her point to register. "Thanks a lot."

"Oh, no, I didn't mean it in a bad way." She put her hand on my knee. "I'm *so sorry*. That didn't come out right. You're fine. I mean, you're normal. You don't need to worry about a thing."

Up until that moment, I hadn't.

There are certain conversations that rattle you to your core. Those two minutes with Beth was one. Now at once the fact that the girl back in Flushing wouldn't leave her fireman boyfriend made total sense. It wasn't because he ran into burning buildings and I . . . well, I didn't run into burning buildings. It was because he had a bigger penis than I did. You don't skip the Eiffel Tower because you're afraid you might miss the Leaning Tower of Pisa.

I left Beth's room shaking my head and reassessing my life.

Clyde was still in his room when I walked back inside. He looked up at me and said, "Well?"

"Congratulations."

"You know, it really *isn't* such a big deal."

"Said the guy who lives with six women."

"Five," he said.

"Depends on the day of the week, right?"

He reached into his shirt pocket. "You want to smoke that joint now?"

I sat down next to him on the couch. "Yeah."

He reached into his pants pocket, pulled out a cigarette lighter, and lit up the joint. He offered it to me first with a kind of ceremonial flourish, a backhand wave that ended in an "okay" sign, with the joint between his thumb and forefinger. But I declined. So he took a long drag, then passed it across the couch in a more matter-of-fact way. "Ready to pop your cherry?"

"Please, don't put it like that," I said.

He laughed, and I took a quick puff.

"Don't let the smoke out," he said.

I kept the smoke in my throat for several seconds, but then exhaled. "Sorry."

"I should've told you to take a deep breath first. Try again."

I breathed in and out hard, then puffed on the joint a second time. This time I was able to hold the smoke much longer, maybe twenty seconds.

"Feel the difference?"

"It's warm," I said.

"That's how it starts."

He and I passed the joint back and forth until it was down to a glowing nub. Then he pulled out a clip, and we smoked the nub down to nothing. Afterward, the back of my throat burned, but otherwise I felt no different. I didn't want to disappoint Clyde, so I stretched out my arms and began to sway back and forth. It was what he did when he got high.

He smiled. "It's like a whole new perspective on things, isn't it?"

"Yeah."

"I know what you're thinking. You're thinking that what you're feeling now isn't reality. But who's to say what's real and what's not? Maybe this is reality, and the way you were feeling a few minutes ago, that's the illusion. I mean, no one really knows, right?"

"What's on the film projector?"

"You ever hear of Bettie Page?"

"No," I said.

"She was a porno actress in the 1950s. You want to watch a couple of her loops?"

"No thanks."

"It's not *porno* porno," he said. "C'mon, it's not even X-rated. It's like a classic."

"I don't know . . ."

"There's no sound, so if you don't like it, you can always just close your eyes."

"Fine," I said.

He leaned forward and switched on the film projector. The light came on, and the film began to roll, and a second later, a flickering black and white image gathered against the bare wall across the room. It turned out I *did* know who Bettie Page was—or at least I recognized her face from magazine photos I'd seen. I thought she was just another B-movie actress from the 1950s. But there she was, cavorting in her underwear, strutting back and forth in a dingy room, and then . . . spanking another woman. Clyde was right. It wasn't *porno* porno. It was just kind of odd.

He was chuckling as he watched. After I couple of minutes, I began to laugh too—not out loud. Just to myself. But also *at* myself, at the fact that I'd traveled three thousand miles to get away from reality, to smoke a joint, and, as it turned out, to discover that my dearest childhood friend had a penis the size of an archipelago. Maybe the marijuana *was* having an effect. But as I watched Bettie Page on that cracked wall, spanking her little heart out, right in the thick of her life, doing what she had to do to get by, I thought about the miles I'd come, about the ride itself, about the one-eyed jacks, about the long passage from Pennsylvania to Ohio, about the happy interlude with Margie, about the brutal stretch of West Texas nothing, about the uncrossed bridge to Juarez, about the taste of sidewalk in Santa Barbara, and I thought about the miles I still had to go, about the ride back to New York, about the ride back to my life, about the girl I loved, who was about to reject me for a fireman.

How could you regret it? How could you regret a moment of it?

WRITING A BESTSELLER

The year I graduated from high school, my father gave me some advice that I've been turning over in my mind ever since. Actually, it wasn't advice so much as a comprehensive assessment combined with an exhortation to act. The fact that it came slathered in Yiddish (and, thus, also in thick morning mucous) made it even more memorable: "*Foyl de aft hundt!*"

The rough translation is: "Lazy like a dog!"

What he meant was, "Get a freakin' job!"

The thing my father didn't understand was that I didn't need to get a job, not at that moment and not in the foreseeable future, because I was a *writer*. Granted, at that moment, I was an unpublished writer. But that was a mere technicality, a point of interest to literary historians perhaps, but even as twelfth grade wound down, I had a pretty detailed image of what the next few years would hold: By the time I graduated college, I would be churning out critically acclaimed novels, getting compared (favorably) with Faulkner, Hemingway, and Fitzgerald, collecting Pulitzers and sipping champagne out of Inger Stevens's slipper. (I should note, parenthetically, that I didn't drink champagne, and that Inger Stevens had, unbeknownst to me, died several years earlier. But even after I learned of her untimely end while flipping through the pages of the 1974 *World Almanac*, I had no doubt that her slippers could still be had for the right price, and anyway, my distaste for champagne, and Inger Stevens's fatal barbiturate overdose, were also mere technicalities, and future Pulitzer Prize-winning writers didn't concern themselves with technicalities, or, for that matter, with parenthetical statements.)

Close parenthesis.

By the time I graduated college, I *was* indeed churning out novels. Three of them. I was churning them out on a secondhand IBM Selectric, keeping my roommate Mitchell awake into the wee hours of the morning, because churning out novels turns out to involve more clacking and dinging than buttery, laborious silence. The moment they were fully churned, I slid them into manila envelopes, addressed them to names I'd picked out of the *Writer's Market '78* and waited for those big advances and multi-book contracts to start rolling in. I waited, and waited, and waited, and waited . . . and if you add about thirty-five more *waited*'s to that list, you'll approximate the number of form-letter rejections I accumulated from major New York publishers.

Clearly, I was ahead of my time.

Seven more years and six more book-length manuscripts came and went, during which I also squeezed in graduate school and adjunct lecturing. John replaced Mitchell, and a Kaypro 16 replaced the IBM Selectric, and still I kept churning and churning, eager for the day when my time would catch up with me. But rejection followed rejection—and that doesn't even take into account the many approximations of Inger Stevens who did not succumb to my genius. Not for a moment, however, did I think of myself as an *aspiring* writer or even a *struggling* writer. I was a writer, dammit, and the fact that my conduit to critical acclaim and wide readership had yet to open was an uncomfortable but short-term predicament, akin to a fecal impaction of novels.

Then, in 1986, I had a moment of clarity: The thing to do was to write a bestseller first, then move on to the more literary Pulitzer Prize-winning stuff. The problem was that I'd never actually *read* a bestseller. So I hopped the 7 train into Manhattan, trekked over to the

Scribner Book Store on Fifth Avenue, and pulled down the first novel from the paperback bestseller rack that caught my eye: *Lie Down With Lions*, by Ken Follett. I opened it at random to page 6 and read: "He looked at her wide mouth, the full lips that kissed him so often and so lusciously."

And I thought: *In a weak moment, I might type, "he looked at her wide mouth," and if you put a gun to my head, maybe even "the full lips that kissed him so often," but under no circumstances were those lips going to be kissing him, or anyone else, "lusciously."*

Whatever I wrote was going to be better than that.

So I decided just to write. Screw Faulkner, Hemingway, and Fitzgerald. Screw the Pulitzer Prize. Screw art. I would write ten pages per day for the next month, which would give me three hundred-plus pages . . . and therefore, by the Law of Ken Follett, a bestseller.

Plot?

What if Middle Eastern terrorists began kidnapping and killing the children of world diplomats?

Characters?

Well, you had to have a guy. That much I knew. So I came up with a CIA agent named Jeremy Edge. Oh, and a beautiful woman. You definitely want one of those. I named her Inger. She was also a CIA operative . . . *or was she*? Also, you had to have a terrorist leader with a scary-sounding nickname. The Eel. Oh, and a title. You need a catchy, faux-erudite title. I came up with *Unpurged Images* . . . from the William Butler Yeats poem "Byzantium."

And I was off . . .

For the first week, I kept to my ten-pages-per-day plan. I soon learned dialogue filled up more pages than description, so Edge and Inger played a lot of cat and mouse, exchanging cryptic comments across desks and coffee tables and, of course, pillows. Also, every page or so, something blew up . . . because "Boom!" can be a paragraph by itself. So cars exploded. Suitcases exploded. Passions exploded.

By the second week, however, I was down to eight pages per day. By the third week, I was down to seven, with an occasional six. Still, even at roughly seven pages per day, I'd have a novel after six weeks if

I could keep it up. Every so often, of course, I'd glance at a few paragraphs of *Lie Down With Lions*—just to make sure what I was writing was still better than what Ken Follett was writing. So, for example, on page 35, K.F. writes: "She knew she was going to have to leave him. She loved him to distraction, but it seemed he could not love her the same way."

That got me through another two weeks.

I hit page 250 on day thirty-one—well above my seven-pages-per-day average. That night, I cracked open Follett again and found this gem: "He felt her come with a long, gentle, wavy Sunday morning orgasm."

Yeah, I was feeling pretty good about myself around then. I was feeling even better when I passed 300 the following week; the manuscript now took up most of the memory on a 5.25-inch floppy disk. Three hundred pages, moreover, was a benchmark. It meant I was almost home; I needed to start winding this bad boy down.

It was at that point that I made a critical decision. Until then, I'd never read more than a few paragraphs of Ken Follett in one sitting. To get a feel for pacing as I put the finishing touches on *Unpurged Images*, I decided to go back and read *Lie Down With Lions* cover to cover.

I opened the book to page 1—the first time I'd seen page 1—on a Thursday night.

I finished the book just before dawn on Saturday.

It was the greatest thing I'd ever read. All those clichés you hear about bestsellers—couldn't put it down . . . couldn't stop turning pages . . . missed my stop on the train—they were all horribly, joyously, lusciously true. I laughed, I cried, I had a Sunday-morning orgasm (on Friday afternoon).

I loved *Lie Down With Lions . . . to distraction.*

Then, sadly, I began to re-read my three hundred pages.

I had three hundred pages of. . .crap. Of unpurged crap.

Was the prose better, line by line, than Ken Follett's? Yeah, probably. Did that matter? Not one iota. I'd written three hundred pages of not-bad prose. Follett had written a novel, a riveting, gut-churning, heart-pounding novel.

Because I'm anal retentive, I finished *Unpurged Images*. I never even bothered to send it out. To this day, the manuscript sits in a manila envelope, inside a cardboard box, on an unreachable upper shelf, in my linen closet.

And no one is looking for it.

MY MALIBU LIFE

My aunt Tillie always looked after me. Even toward the end, when she was half out of her mind, she gave me her car. She'd moved back home to Shreveport after forty-five years on the Upper East Side of Manhattan and, through a Book of Revelation-level coincidence of unlikelihoods, had passed her road test and gotten her first driver's license at the tender age of sixty-seven. She paid cash for a brand-new '79 Chevy Malibu—whereupon she began a protracted assault on the trees of Louisiana. She would pull out of her driveway, see a car a hundred yards away, and swerve violently to avoid it. All told, she hit six trees. She never hit them hard, never uprooted a single one, but she filed six separate insurance claims . . . at which point the state of Louisiana, perhaps at the behest of the local arboreal society, asked that she no longer drive within its jurisdiction.

So she gave me her Malibu. She hired a guy who did such things to drive it from Shreveport to Flushing, Queens. He showed up in front of my apartment building a week later, reeking of pot, and handed me the deed of sale (for one dollar, which I never made good on), the registration, and two sets of keys. The car still had dead leaves and chads of dried-out bark in the windshield wiper bays.

Still, tooling around downtown Flushing that afternoon, I was overcome by a sudden intoxicating sense of *mine-ness*. Not only did I own the car, I owned the space inside the car . . it was utterly and unequivocally mine. Plus, it *moved*. If it started to rain, and I was miles from home, I would stay dry because I was in the space I owned inside my car. Oh, and the trunk! It was like another closet. And, by the way, it *moved*. If I stuffed it with . . . stuff, and if I drove it miles from home, when I arrived and cracked it open, my stuff would be there.

That first week, however, my education began in the hard realities of owning a car in downtown Flushing. For example, parking on the street was a no-go. Though I was quite the parallel parker as a teenager, back in the neighborhoodly calm of Thirty-Fourth Avenue, when I'd borrow my mother's Rambler on Saturday nights to chauffeur around my nerd herd, finding a space on the street for the Malibu in downtown Flushing was like punching in a higher weight class. A legal spot opened up about once every half life of uranium . . . and when it did, even if you saw it, and even if you were willing to make a quick U-turn into oncoming traffic to beat out the other twelve drivers eyeballing the space, alternate-side-of-the-street rules meant you had to wake up crack-of-early the next morning to move the car again. So, in the end, I shelled out seventy-five dollars per month—roughly one-third of my apartment rent—for Space #33 in the underground garage of my building.

Imagine, then, my annoyance several weeks into my new Malibu life when I drove home just before midnight, rolled into the garage . . . and found Space #33 occupied by a silver-gray Mercury Monarch.

I pulled up behind the Monarch, stepped out of the Malibu, and just stared. For a full minute, I stared in disbelief at the rear bumper of the Monarch. After that, I worked myself up to a couple of fist shakes, the kind of comically broad gestures mimes make to let the entire audience know they're mad. Except there was no audience. Only me and several dozen unoccupied cars in the harsh fluorescent light of the garage. Space #33, my seventy-five-dollar-per-month *private* parking space, was taken. I'd been put out. Usurped. Cuckolded. It was an indignity, an outright indignity, and I was indignant. I considered parking in the nearest open space, but that would serve only to pay the indignity forward. So I decided to absorb it, to park the Malibu out on the street. It was a "*What would Jesus do?*" moment decades before that slogan caught on—decades, in fact, before the slogan "*Pay it forward*" caught on.

I drove out of the garage and searched the boulevards and avenues for the next half hour until at last I found a not-quite-legal-but-maybe-no-one-will-notice-how-close-I-am-to-this-fire-hydrant spot almost a mile from my apartment. During the long walk home, I was filled, once again, with indignation. More than indignation. Righteous indignation. Where was Justice? Where was God? Why do bad things happen to good people?

Exhaustion overcame me when I got back home, and I plopped down on my beat-up convertible sofa. The worn-out mattress coils greeted me with their familiar lunar twang, and I tried to settle in for the night, but it's never a good idea to go to bed with a theodicy stuck in your craw. I couldn't fall asleep. I couldn't get over the fact that I'd been done dirt, and that somewhere in my building the dirt-doer was sleeping soundly. So at three in the morning I climbed out of bed, sat down at my desk, and began to type:

> *To whom it may concern:*
>
> *You don't know me. I'm no one to you. Nothing more than a doormat to be carelessly stepped on, or a parking space to be casually taken. But I am someone. I'm the guy who had to drive around and around the neighborhood for an hour, after midnight, to find a parking space on the street because your car was in Space #33, which I rent each month. How do I rent it, you ask? With hard-earned money. But it did me no good last night, did it? So now, I'm the guy who'll have to wake up early in the morning to walk a mile and move the car to avoid a parking ticket because it's on the wrong side of the street. I'm sure you're thinking, "Well, them's the breaks." And I guess you're right, in a sense. But what kind of world would it be if everyone thought like that?*
>
> *Sincerely, Space #33*

After I'd typed up the note, I headed downstairs and slipped it under the windshield wiper of the Monarch. Then I came back upstairs and slept like a baby.

The next morning, when I went downstairs to check, the Monarch was gone. I felt relief, but also satisfaction imagining the shame the driver must have experienced when he read my note. There was a lightness in my step as I retrieved the Malibu from the woolly outskirts of south Flushing and brought it back to its secure and rightful home. I sighed as I turned off the ignition. As I slammed shut the driver's door, the metallic chunk echoed with finality. The ordeal was over. The car had never looked more fitted to its spot, equidistant between the two yellow lines of Space #33.

Resolution was mine.

But the following day there was a note folded up and pinned under my windshield wiper. I had a bad feeling in my gut as I reached for it; the feeling got worse as I unfolded the paper and began to read:

Dear 33,

I'm so sorry for taking your spot. I got confused. I was looking for 37. I must've parked there a million times. I wasn't myself last night. My son got killed. He got robbed coming home from work. He got killed. I thought 33 was 37. I wasn't paying attention. I'm very sorry. I didn't mean to do it. I apologize. It wont happen again.

Sincerely, 37

It was no bluff. The handwriting was barely legible. Whoever had written it was emotionally and spiritually broken. That much was clear. I read the note over and over and thought about the note I'd written, and I felt sick to my stomach.

I must have drafted half a dozen apologies, but in the end none of them sufficed. I did the only thing I could think to do: I left a sympathy card underneath the windshield wiper of Space #37 and prayed I'd never have to look him in the eye. I never did. Several weeks later, the Mercury Monarch was gone from Space #37.

* * *

As shameful as that moment was, it was soon eclipsed by the day-to-day advantages of owning a car in New York City. Come summer, I began driving to Manhattan on Sunday mornings to play softball—a great luxury, since it meant I no longer had to haul a twenty-pound backpack of sports gear and paraphernalia on the subway.

The games started at nine o'clock, but I liked to arrive an hour beforehand to begin the extended ritual of hamstring stretching, light tossing and ointment application before stepping out onto the field. Factor in a forty-five minute drive to Central Park, and another forty-five minutes to find a parking space (again!), and I was leaving the house around six-thirty. But one particular Sunday, as I recall, I got an earlier-than-usual start. It was the third week in August, and my bedroom was sweltering, so rather than lie in bed sweating, I figured I'd head out to softball at six; if nothing else, parking would be easier.

By six fifteen, I was driving north along the Grand Central Parkway when I realized I had to pee. Not a problem. I come from a long line of weak-bladdered Semites, and, even in my twenties, I knew the nearest public restroom anywhere and anytime I was likely to be predisposed. I calmly exited the highway and pulled into the parking lot of the Hampton Inn by LaGuardia Airport. In short order, I found the men's room on the deserted mezzanine level and did what I came to do. But as I was about to leave, I heard a commotion at the far end of the hall . . . a pimp was roughing up a prostitute.

The swing and clack of the men's room door caught both of their attentions.

"Look at that!" the prostitute shouted. "You ain't going to do shit!"

The pimp glared at me. "You just keep right on walking, my man . . ."

"No, you stay right here," the prostitute said. "You be my witness."

"Hey, I'm not looking for trouble," I said, still at a safe distance.

The pimp grinned slyly. "Then I suggest you keep on walking."

I didn't move.

"What did I tell you?" the prostitute shouted. "He's a witness."

The pimp shoved her against the wall, then took a step toward me. "You a witness?"

"I'm not a witness," I said.

"There—"

"But I see what's going on."

"I thought you said you're not a witness."

"I'm *not* a witness," I said. "But I *do* see what's going on."

He held out his hands, palms upward. "What's the difference?"

"You know what the difference is."

"You're either a witness or not a witness. Ain't no in-between."

"I disagree."

"You can't disagree," he said. "It's either-or."

I shrugged. "Then I guess we're kind of stuck."

The prostitute began to laugh. "You better watch it, Jamal. That's one crazy-ass white boy. He's liable to shoot both of us just for the hell of it."

The pimp looked me up and down. "Nah, he ain't gonna do nothing."

"I don't know," she said. "He got that crazy-ass white-boy look, like he's been talking to dogs."

They were both laughing at that point, and I was smiling at the fact that they were laughing.

"You can move along now," the prostitute said.

"Are you sure?"

The pimp nodded. "G'on, get your crazy ass out of here."

The peaceable kingdom seemed to be restored, so I left.

Flushing, during the mid-1980s, was undergoing an ethnic upheaval. What had, for most of my life, been a largely white, middle-class enclave was being drastically transformed by wave after wave of immigration from Asia. Chinese, Japanese, Vietnamese, Thai, and Korean families arrived in huddled masses, settling within walking distance of the Main Street subway station, bringing with them exotic foods, unreadable signage, and the many cultural mysteries of the Orient, including an unreasoning passion for Rockport sandals.

It was during this time that the comic stereotype of the bad Asian driver began to gain traction. (Andrew Dice Clay, as I recall, had much to say, and much of it offensive, on the subject.) It was, of course, true, and my 'hood was the unofficial epicenter of traffic inscrutability. Not every Asian driver in Flushing was an outright menace, but the percentage reached critical mass, and soon enough even a short trip up Kissena Boulevard to Queens College evolved into a vehicular gauntlet the likes of which would have set Mario Andretti's teeth on edge.

My response, from behind the wheel of my Malibu, was to "turtle up." Turtling up, in the vernacular of professional hockey, is a preemptive response to an imminent threat: You fall to the ice on your stomach and cover your vulnerable points in order to avoid getting your brains bashed in. Translated into driving, *turtling up* means hypervigilance; it means following the letter of the law, right down to signaling each lane change, obeying the posted speed limit, and bracing for whiplash at every stop sign.

Thus, in the late afternoon of December 18, 1986, I rolled to an unsudden stop behind a line of cars to await the left-turn signal on College Point Boulevard at Roosevelt Avenue. Another car pulled up behind me, but didn't rear-end me, so I exhaled and began to fuss with the radio. Just as I lucked into a Beatles song, "Lady Madonna," I heard a siren. Not a siren, exactly. It was one of those terse bleats that police cars emit in lieu of an actual siren. Naturally, I looked up, glanced around. The police car had been headed in the opposite direction and had pulled over against the opposite curb. So I had no idea who'd done what. Nothing happened for several moments. Then, from the lane to my right, a beat-up green car the size of a tugboat eased over toward the sidewalk. And I grinned: He deserved a ticket for driving a car that ugly! But while I pondered the proper fine for bad aesthetics, the police car bleated again. Again I glanced around, looking for another ugly car. Then came a third bleat, this one even terser than the first two—the sound, I swear, was sarcastic. Still, nothing was happening. So I looked over again at the ugly green car, but it hadn't moved.

Then came the cop's voice, on the loudspeaker: "Pull over!"

I looked at him and thought, *Gee, if I didn't know better I'd swear he was talking to me . . .*

So I flashed him a cartoon "who, me?" gesture, to which he replied, again on the loudspeaker: "Yes, you!"

All right, I thought. No reason to panic. Maybe he's got a report of a stolen Malibu. So I pulled out of the left-turn lane and eased up behind the ugly green car. Not where I wanted to be, but I was in no rush. The police car made a U-turn to come up behind me. I waited as the cop walked past me, without a word, and approached the driver's side of the green car. As he did, the driver began to climb out of his car. The cop shouted at him to stay in his car, but the man got out anyway. He was a well-dressed Asian man, perhaps in his late forties. The cop spoke to him for about three minutes; there were severe language problems and much hand-waving on both sides. Afterward, the Asian man got back in his car and drove off.

Then the cop, a husky guy who looked to be in his mid-twenties, walked back to me, leaned over my window, and said, "License and registration."

I fished out my license from my wallet and the car registration from the glove compartment. As I handed them to the cop, I looked up and said, as meekly as I could, "May I ask why?"

"You ran that red light back there."

"What light?"

"Back there." He pointed. "One block."

"No I didn't," I said.

"You followed the green car through it."

"But I was already in the left-turn lane. I got here before the green car."

He smiled at me. "Hey, guy, I wouldn't give you a ticket for nothing."

Except then he did.

Naturally, I filled out the back of the summons and pleaded Not Guilty. I really and truly *hadn't* run the red light, and I damn sure wasn't going to pay a fifty-dollar fine for something I hadn't done. What I couldn't figure out was why the cop had ticketed me in the first place. I kept going over the sequence of events, and a week before the trial, I thought I'd figured it out. The cop had spotted the ugly green car run the red light, and then, out of the corner of his eye, he must have noticed another car follow. But as he strained to keep the green car in sight, he must have become confused between the second car and mine. That was my Second Car Hypothesis, upon which I planned to rest my defense. I was pretty confident.

February 2 was my trial date. Friends offered all kinds of advice: "Wear a suit. It shows respect for the court." "Don't wear a suit. It looks too confident." "Be forceful." "Be humble." "Look the judge in the eyes." "Never look the judge in the eyes." In the end, I decided to dress for work—a tie but no suit—and hope for the best.

When I arrived at the Hearing Office, I was directed to Room 2, which turned out to be a miniature courtroom. For an hour, I sat on a slick wooden bench as drivers confronted their uniformed accusers and pleaded their causes. The very first case was thrown out because the cop had failed to write up the ticket properly. After that came a string of convictions, all of which seemed to me justified. One guy, accused of running a red light, claimed it had been yellow, then claimed it had been broken, then claimed he wasn't on the street in the first place. It turned out to be his third conviction in six months, and his license was suspended.

Finally, my name was called. The cop from that fateful day approached the bench, and we stood before the judge side by side. He smiled at me. Clearly, there were no hard feelings. He swore to tell the truth, and he methodically recited the account from his notepad. He said he witnessed my car follow a green Oldsmobile through a steady red on College Point Boulevard, ascertained that the signal was in working order, and then issued a summons to both cars.

"Two cars went through the signal?" the judge asked him.

"Yes."

"And you saw them both?"

I interrupted, "That's my point, your honor."

"You'll have your turn in a minute," the judge snapped at me, then turned back to the cop: "Two cars drove through the signal, and you never lost sight of either one?"

Way to go, judgy! I thought: *Shadow of a doubt! Shadow of a doubt!*

"No sir," the cop said.

Now it was my turn: I swore to tell the truth and recounted what had happened, right down to "Lady Madonna." Then I explained my Second Car Hypothesis, at which both the judge and the cop smiled. It was very friendly. Recalling that a ticket-quota scandal had hit the papers the day before, I added that I thought it was an honest mistake, that the officer had been courteous. *No reason to cast aspersions*, I thought.

"Anything else?" the judge asked.

It occurred to me to compliment his tie, but I decided against it. "No, your honor."

Now the judge looked me square in the eyes: "I find that the officer has sustained his case, and I order you to pay the fifty-dollar fine plus seventeen-dollar surcharge. Do you have the money with you?"

Stunned, I nodded yes.

"Pay the cashier on the way out."

Forking over the sixty-seven dollars took a toll not only on my wallet but on my psychic attachment to the Malibu. Yeah, the thing kept me dry in the rain. Yeah, it held my stuff. But it also seemed to underscore the capriciousness of life. You could be in the right, but wind up wrong. You could be brave, but in a cowardly way. You could follow the rules, but still be fined.

No doubt, I was overthinking it. But wasn't that fact, in itself, an indication that I shouldn't own a car? Overthinking and driving are a bad combination. I'm guessing more accidents result from ruminative driving than from drunk driving. Think of it this way: Who would you rather have take you to the airport when you're running late? A lit crit professor or a cabbie?

Maybe I wasn't car-owner material . . .

The point became moot a couple of years later when I moved into Midtown Manhattan. I realized I couldn't afford to keep both the Malibu and myself in the city—the rent for garage space was roughly equal to what I was paying for my apartment in Flushing.

On the day I sold the Malibu to a friend of mine, for the price of a steak dinner, I circled the car one last time to inspect its condition (but really to say a secret goodbye, and mumble an apology under my breath). As I made my way around to the front, I found an inch-long strip of tree bark still lodged in the windshield wiper bay.

I left it there.

SAUL BELLOW OWES ME A FAVOR

Saul Bellow died owing me a favor. He never knew it, or I'm sure he would have tracked me down and thanked me, heartily, and perhaps even treated me like a son, but the universe knew it, in the way the universe knows things, and thus, many years after the fact, Bellow's son Adam read a column of mine, tracked me down, and asked me to write a book for him at HarperCollins, where he was an editor.

But I've gotten ahead of myself.

It was the fall of 1982, and I'd just begun graduate school. Pragmatic as always, I had enrolled in the MA program in creative writing at Queens College. My first class was a fiction workshop with the literary critic Robert Towers. Now regrettably obscure, Towers was a big cheese at the time. He wrote front-page reviews for the Sunday *Times Book Review*, the kind of reviews that made authors' careers. He looked the part too. Broad through the chest and gut, with horn-rimmed glasses and a shock of thick gray hair, he was rumpled to a comical degree; his suit pants couldn't have held a crease if they'd been pressed for millions years by a force equal to plate tectonics. Clearly, he had things besides ironing on his mind. Literary things. He was easily the most eminent guy I'd ever met, and of course I wanted to impress him with my writing. More than that, I wanted to impress him with *me*. I wanted him to like me, to look forward to chatting with me, to nod approvingly at my opinions about literature. The problem was that I had no opinions about literature, or at least none that were likely to gain approving nods. When it came to literature, I had less an aesthetic sense than a targeted narcolepsy. If the first few pages of a book didn't lull me into REM sleep, I could usually keep going until the end. That was what I brought to the table, my entire critical apparatus.

But I *did* have a car, a 1979 Chevy Malibu. The fact that I had a car mattered because Robert Towers didn't. He lived on the Upper West Side of Manhattan and had to take a train and then a bus to Queens College. Which meant he was not only an eminent guy; he was an eminent guy in need of a lift to the subway.

So one drizzly Wednesday night I stayed in my seat as the rest of the students filed out of the classroom. I was looking down, pretending to scribble in my spiral notebook, and then I looked up, pretending to be startled that he and I were the only two people left in the room. I said, "It's raining outside. I've got a car. Do you need a ride anywhere?"

"Thanks, but I live in Manhattan," he said, smiling. "I couldn't ask you to—"

"How about if I drop you off at the subway station in Forest Hills? That way you won't have to wait in the rain for the bus."

Thus began a weekly ritual.

For the first few Wednesdays, we spoke about my writing . . . about the short stories I'd handed in, about the new ones I was working on, about the novels I was sketching out (even as I steered the Malibu down Jewel Avenue). It was during the third week, as I recall, that he asked me which current writers I admired.

"Well, um, I'm partial to . . . I mean, it's hard to say. There are so many!"

"Yes, I agree," he said. "There are riches to choose from."

"I mean, obviously, there's Faulkner and Hemingway and Fitzgerald."

"But among *current* writers, do you have a favorite?"

I let out a knowing laugh, which I wasn't sure I could carry off. "It's like choosing my favorite Beatles song. As soon as I mention one, I'm going to think of five others I like more."

"I see your point," he said.

I doubted he did . . . unless he was referring to the figurative dunce cap on top of my head. Luckily, at that moment, we arrived at the subway station in Forest Hills, and he climbed out of the car.

"I'll see you next week," I called after him.

He waved back at me.

I felt like a—*what's the right word?*—dunce.

I pulled away from the curb, however, with a newfound purpose. I would become conversant in contemporary American prose. Preferably by the following Wednesday. The next morning, I drove to the Brentano's bookstore in the Queens Center mall and made a beeline for the reference section. It was there, in the far-right corner of the very bottom shelf, that I discovered Martin Seymour Smith's *Who's Who in Twentieth Century Literature.*

It was an encyclopedia, only nastier. Smith was opinionated, and he was merciless. The entry for Ernest Hemingway begins, "American fiction writer, traveler, journalist, hunter and killer of animals, perpetrator of semi-accurate reminiscence." Of William Burroughs, Smith writes, "He is a spoiled child, mildly funny when dealing with the most obvious deficiencies of the modern world, but mostly an exploiter of his own obsessions with homosexuality, violence and policemen. His prose style, where one can get at it, is undistinguished." And pity poor Sinclair Lewis: "[He] is only of socio-anthropological interest; as a writer, he is almost worthless . . ."

I lived with the book for the next week, highlighting in yellow Smith's most brutal takedowns, highlighting in blue the authors Smith thought merely overrated, and highlighting in green (by highlighting in both yellow and blue) the handful of authors Smith deemed worthy of their human ingredients. I was too vain to pass off Smith's judgments as my own, or even to pretend I'd read what I hadn't—besides, I'd watched enough sitcoms to know how those conversations ended—but at least I'd have a few names to throw around: "*Well, you know, I haven't read him myself, but I've heard interesting things about . . .*"

My weeklong cram had the desired effect. The next Wednesday, Bob Towers and I were batting names back and forth like Chinese Ping-Pong players. He was supplying the speed and spin of course; I was only blocking the ball back into his court. ("I've always thought of Updike as a *New Yorker* writer. I mean, it's obviously true in the literal sense. But do you think that's too limiting?") Still, it was a glorious fifteen-minute drive. Toward the end, he told me he'd been asked to review Saul Bellow's new novel, *The Dean's December*. It was Bellow's first since he'd been awarded the Nobel Prize, so the assignment was quite a coup. Towers asked me if I'd read Bellow's previous novel, *Humboldt's Gift*. Since we were only a block from the subway station, and he was about to get out of the car, I risked the teensiest of lies.

"Actually," I said, "I just started it a couple of days ago."

"Ah!"

"I mean, I'm only a little ways in—"

"Well, you must tell me your thoughts when you finish."

The first thing I did when I got home was look up Saul Bellow in *Who's Who in Twentieth Century Literature*—I wanted to get Martin Seymour Smith's take on the guy before I went out and bought *Humboldt's Gift*. Smith was decidedly lukewarm: "Bellow has become increasingly victim to the fatal notion of the 'Great American Novel', but has been driven to this not by ambition but by his delicate, humorous sensibility and his passionate and frustrated desire to produce an answer to the twin nihilisms of mindless leftist extremism and faceless bureaucracy." (I understood about half of that.) On the other hand, Smith called the ending of Bellow's novel *Seize the Day* "one of the most moving passages in modern literature," and, more to the point, he called *Humboldt's Gift* "a return to form."

The next morning, I plunked down three ninety-nine at Brentano's for a paperback copy of *Humboldt's Gift*.

Let me be the first to admit it. Much of the book, the first time through, went right over my head. The literary gossip, the lectures in theosophy, the creaky Yiddishisms . . . I had no clue what Bellow was getting at. But the writing! The rhythm of the sentences, the cascading metaphors, the slapstick one-liners . . . I'd never read anything like it. It didn't even feel like reading a book. It felt more like having an uncle sit you down and tell you stories about the way things were when he was your age (if your uncle happened to be exceptionally smart, exceptionally funny, and occasionally cranky).

Even Bellow's character descriptions were chiseled and cut like jewels. Here's the narrator of *Humboldt's Gift*, Charlie Citrine, recalling his long-deceased lover, Demmie Vonghel:

> But in a few minutes I heard what I expected to hear—her night voice. It was low hoarse and deep, almost mannish. She moaned. She spoke in broken words. She did this almost every night. The voice expressed her terror of this strange place, the earth, and of this strange state, being. Laboring and groaning she tried to get out of it. This was the primordial Demmie beneath the farmer's daughter beneath the teacher beneath the elegant Main Line horsewoman, Latinist, accomplished cocktail-sipper in black chiffon, with the upturned nose, this fashionable conversationalist . . .

Bellow was doing things with language I didn't know language could do. When I finished *Humboldt's Gift* several days later, I wanted to rip up every page I'd ever written and become a longshoreman. (My preternatural scrawniness argued against it, however.) But at least I had a definite opinion on the subject of Saul Bellow, an opinion I'd derived the old-fashioned way—by, like, you know, reading an actual book—so I'd be able to hold up my end of the front-seat conversation with Towers during our next ride to Forest Hills. The problem was that I didn't want to gush. I wanted to say something more insightful than, *Saul Bellow? I just love him. He's so good. He's just soooo good. The way he writes. I mean he's just soooo good. I want to hang his poster over my bed and start a fan club and maybe marry him someday.*

What I needed was a formulated phrase.

After a couple of false starts—"Bellow well-deserved the recognition of the Nobel Committee" and "The tradition of the novel of ideas is in good hands"—I came up with what felt like a passable line: "Sentence by sentence, Bellow is simply the best writer we have."

I said it to myself several times; it sounded erudite yet straightforward, the kind of thing you could plausibly improvise if you were given to weighty intellectual judgments. I especially liked the "we"—as in, "we erudite folks who are given to weighty intellectual judgments."

I tried it out the next morning on my roommate, Mitchell. "You know, I just finished *Humboldt's Gift*, and I have to say, sentence by sentence, Saul Bellow is simply the best writer we have."

He closed the refrigerator. "We're out of cream cheese."

"I'll go to the grocery store later. But don't you think that sentence by sentence, Bellow is simply the best writer we have?"

He stared at me. "Are you drunk?"

"Why? Who do you think is better?"

"I don't know," he said. "Why are we having this conversation?"

"I told you. I just finished *Humboldt's Gift* . . ."

He walked back into his room, shaking his head.

So I phoned my friend Phil and tried out the line on him.

There was a long pause on the other end. "You mean that Bellow is the best writer, sentence by sentence, in America. Is that right?"

"Yes."

"But not necessarily the best writer in the English language, right? There could be writers who are better than Bellow, sentence by sentence, in Great Britain or Australia, right?"

"No."

"So what you're saying is that, sentence by sentence, Bellow is the best writer currently writing in the English language . . . the same way Sugar Ray Robinson was, pound for pound, the best fighter in the world."

"Well, when you say it that way, it sounds kind of stupid."

"It *is* kind of stupid. How would you even make that call?"

"I told you. I just finished *Humboldt's Gift*—"

"Did Bellow knock out Salinger in the twelfth chapter?"

Phil was still laughing as I hung up the phone. But the more I thought about it, the more determined I was to stand by my judgment. Critics say things all the time that carry great import but don't quite hold up to logical analysis. (Wines aren't *really* "insouciant," if you stop and think about it.) So I had my formulated phrase. I looked forward, mixed-metaphorically speaking, to running it up the flagpole and seeing if Robert Towers saluted.

That opportunity came, as I'd hoped, after class the following Wednesday night. Towers asked me how I was liking *Humboldt's Gift* as we came to a traffic light on Jewel Avenue. I brought the car to a gentle halt, turned to him, and said, "You know, I think it's his finest work . . . which is saying a lot because, *ahem*, sentence by sentence, Bellow is simply the best writer we have."

Towers nodded. "I quite agree."

After I dropped him off at the subway station, in the hundred or so times I replayed his response in my mind, I lingered more and more on the word *quite*. Robert Towers, eminent literary critic, didn't just agree with my assessment of Bellow. He *quite* agreed. I felt vindicated, on a metaphysical level.

Quite vindicated.

It was a couple of months later, and I was sitting in the kitchen, swallowing the last bite of an unfrosted cherry Pop-Tart, debating whether to have another, when the phone rang. The voice at the other end was Phil. The first words out of his mouth were, "You stole that line!"

I pulled the receiver away from my ear and stared at it.

Phil's voice got louder. "Hello? Hello?"

"What are you talking about?" I asked.

"That line about Saul Bellow. You remember, "sentence by sentence . . ."

"I didn't steal that."

"You did too," he said. "You stole that line from Robert Towers."

"He was my professor last semester. But I didn't steal that line—"

"It's in the paper," he said.

"What paper?"

"The Sunday *Times*. Do you have today's paper?"

"It's in the hallway. I haven't brought in it in yet."

"Look on page 22 of the Book Review," he said, "the last paragraph."

Now my curiosity was piqued. I hung up the phone, walked to the front door and opened it, but there was no sign of the paper. I glanced down the hallway in both directions, then shut the door. As I turned around, Mitchell was coming out of his room, waving the Book Review section.

"You've got to read this!" he said.

He handed it to me. It was opened to page 22.

I scanned down to the last paragraph of Robert Towers's review of Saul Bellow's *The Dean's December*. It read:

> *The Dean's December* confirms me in the opinion I have held since, nearly 30 years ago, I read The Adventures of Augie March (having, as an impecunious instructor, paid out hard cash for my hardcover copy just off the press): Sentence by sentence, page by page, Saul Bellow is simply the best writer we have.

I read the paragraph twice, then looked up.

"Towers stole your line," Mitchell said.

"He didn't *steal* my line."

"You said it to me. I remember the 'sentence by sentence' thing."

"Look," I said. "I'm sure he didn't mean to do it. We were talking, and he agreed with me. He probably didn't remember who said what when he was writing the review. It's not a big deal."

"You should sue him!"

"For what?"

"Plagiarism!"

"C'mon, you can't plagiarize a conversation."

"But he used your exact words," Mitchell said. "I'll be your witness."

"He didn't use my *exact* words. He added *page by page*."

"You think that makes a difference? It's still your quote!"

"Forget about it," I said. "Oh, and we need to buy more Pop-Tarts."

I spent the rest of the day, as I did most winter Sundays, playing touch football, watching professional football, and dining out with friends. I thought, intermittently, and without great concern, about the fact that my formulated phrase had made it into the *New York Times* Book Review. It seemed a kind of brush with fame. I was content with the outcome.

The following Friday, however, I was awakened from a dream of Pop-Tarts and football when Mitchell flung *The New York Times* into my bedroom. The thing slapped down on the hardwood floor about a foot from my bed.

"C-27," he called to me.

I rolled out of bed, picked up the paper, and opened it to Section C, page 27.

It was a full-page ad for Saul Bellow's new novel, *The Dean's December*. It had a photo of the author, looking jaunty in a sport jacket and tie, smiling his trademark gap-toothed smile. His face was positioned to the right of a single quotation: "Saul Bellow is simply the best writer that we have."

There was also an insert in the lower-left corner: "See Saul Bellow on Dick Cavett next Monday, Tuesday and Wednesday at 11:00PM on WNET."

"What do you think *now*?" Mitchell called from the kitchen.

"I think it doesn't matter," I called back.

Truth be told, however, I was kind of peeved at that point. For the first time, I considered stopping by Towers's office and asking if he recalled our conversation. But to what end? Even if he did recall it, and even if he apologized sincerely and profusely, what would I have accomplished? Were the editors at the Book Review going to print a correction? What, exactly, did they need to correct? Towers *did* think that Bellow was America's finest writer . . . sentence by sentence. Not only did he think it, he *quite* thought it.

Was a moment's satisfaction—and that was the best-case scenario—worth making a nice man feel bad?

Again, I decided to let it go.

The following Monday, of course, I tuned in to *The Dick Cavett Show* to watch the first installment of Bellow's three-part interview. I'd never even heard the guy's voice; I was anxious to find out what he had to say about writing, about literature, and about life. I leaned forward as Cavett jogged onto the stage. The first words out of his mouth were, "My guest today, Saul Bellow, has been called, 'sentence by sentence, simply the best writer we have' . . ."

"Did you hear that?" Mitchell called from his room.

"Yeah," I said, as much to myself as to him.

I remember little of the interview. What I do remember, as I watched Bellow hold forth on various topics, was the sudden realization that Saul Bellow, winner of the Nobel Prize for literature, winner of the Pulitzer Prize and National Book Award, lover of many beautiful women and serial husband, Saul Bellow, *sentence by sentence, simply the best writer we have*, owed me a favor.

Even if he never knew it. And that ain't nothing.

THE ENCOUNTER

I was in my early thirties when I moved from a spacious one-bedroom apartment in Queens to a cramped studio at the edge of Herald Square in Midtown Manhattan. The idea was to shorten the commute to work. The move itself was hassle-free; I didn't have much furniture, so a couple of softball buddies and I did the entire job in just one trip in a rented, dented U-Haul.

Those first few days were a whirlwind of nesting activities: filling the refrigerator with frozen foods, buying the first microwave I'd ever owned, stocking up on household supplies from the half dozen Duane Reades located within three square blocks of my house, acquiring a new phone line and 212 number, making an appointment with the cable-TV guy, opening an account with Con Edison, tending to the stigmata left by "partial assembly required" furniture.

After a week, I threw myself a housewarming party. Among the towel sets, coffee mugs, and prehensile oven mitts with which my friends warmed my new apartment came a single anonymous gift:

A can of roach spray.

Someone had wrapped it in a liquor box and slipped it amid the pile of presents. No one would own up to the deed afterward. I didn't think much of it at the time, just a gag gift, an inside joke about city living that had nothing to do with me because I kept a clean house.

Still, I was drawn back to the gift once my guests had left. This was not your run-of-the-mill can of insect spray, no cartoon roaches in derby hats playing poker. This was deep blue and serious, a silhouette of the Manhattan skyline below the logo: Special City Formula II. I scoffed at this. Hey, I'd grown up in the *boroughs*: I'd confronted the gangland roaches of Brooklyn, the war-torn vermin of the South Bronx, the Gangpae beetles of Little Korea that seeped in and out of Hefty bags behind restaurants on Roosevelt Avenue. Nevertheless, as I spoke the words out loud, I felt slightly uneasy: *Special City Formula II.* How had Formula I gone awry? The reverse side of the can was striped with minuscule print underneath the italic title: *Precautionary Statements—Hazards To Humans And Domestic Animals.* The hundred or so words consisted of reasons and occasions *not* to use the spray. Its use, the label implied, would set in motion a sequence of events that fell somewhere between extreme unpleasantness and Mutual Assured Destruction.

Still, as I say, I kept a clean house. Oh, sure, I'd seen a couple of roaches that first week before the housewarming. They appeared in tandem as I unpacked the last of a dozen boxes of paperback books. Tokens left over from the last tenant, I figured. Besides, they were such wee things; they had the look of accidental tourists, scurrying futilely across vast expanses of bare white wall toward a sudden shroud of Kleenex.

As I stored my new can of roach spray beneath the bathroom sink, in other words, I never expected to use it.

The Tuesday night following the housewarming, however, I was awakened just after midnight by a rustling sound. It was barely loud enough to stir me, and I wouldn't have gotten out of my newly assembled platform bed except that I couldn't figure out the source. Naturally, the thought of a roach crossed my mind. But I ruled it out; the sound was too substantial. Things were being *moved* in my closet.

So I got out of bed and walked, barefoot, toward the closet. The room was gray under the darkness. Suddenly, the sound stopped; I stopped. Then it started up again . . . except now I thought I knew what it was; I'd received a basket of fragrant scarab soaps at the party, but since I'm not a fragrant-scarab-soap kind of guy, I had afterward tossed the whole business onto a high shelf in the closet. One of the soaps must have come loose and begun to slide down the plastic garment bags hanging below. I threw open the closet doors, and sure enough a scarab soap-sized object dropped to the floor between my feet.

Then it scampered across my left foot and into the bathroom.

Instantly, I passed from half-asleep to awake-enough-to-coordinate-the-combined-air-and-sea-invasion-of-Normandy. I switched on the bathroom light, and there, between the toilet and the tub, he was. He made no effort to hide. There was no place he could have hidden. He was the biggest thing I'd ever seen on six legs. He was like something out of the La Brea Tar Pits, or, better yet, like something out of an old black and white animated short, where he might grab a megaphone and begin to sing like Rudy Vallee. Within that first instant, still, disbelief got the better of terror. I said out loud, "Oh come on!"

That was when terror set in.

This was more than a roach. This was a Presence. This was a great brown sneer disguised as a bug. If Kafka's Gregor Samsa had awakened on the beach, that morning he found himself transformed into a gigantic insect, this thing would have kicked sand in his face. I started to tremble and then, very slowly, backed out of the bathroom.

I leaned against the wall and caught my breath. A trickle of sweat slipped down my spine, and, as it did, my heart jumped to my throat. Now I glanced across the apartment to a distant closet. Where I kept my softball bat.

But then I remembered the roach spray—the deep blue can underneath the bathroom sink.

So I leaned around the edge of the wall and peered back into the bathroom. The roach hadn't moved. That annoyed me. There was an arrogance about it, about the fact that he hadn't moved an inch even though he knew I'd seen him. The natural order of things demanded that he seek cover—even if there was none. He should have at least made the effort. Anger steeled my nerves. Without stepping into the bathroom, and also without taking my eye off the roach, I leaned inside and pulled open the cabinet beneath the sink. The cabinet door creaked loudly, but the roach did not flinch. He only continued to observe me with a certain haughty indifference. He did not seem fazed even by the sight of the deep blue can. Now *that* worried me. If what I was about to do did not kill him, it was certainly going to piss him off. But as I aimed the nozzle in his direction, I had a better idea. Since I did not want him to flee the bathroom after I started to spray—and I surely was not going to get in his way if he bolted—I decided to saturate the floor at the threshold of the bathroom. That way, at least, he would be inclined to run in the opposite direction, where he would hit the side of the bathtub. A dead end. Finally, with great trepidation, I began to spray into the floor at my feet. The fumes were dazzling. Every time I glanced back up at the roach, he seemed to change colors. Brown to blue to deep red. Actually, the deep red became him. He looked like a cinnamon scarab soap. But then my senses cleared, and I trained the nozzle on him.

The first stream of poison sent him staggering backward. He reeled in circles, several of his legs gone limp, a kind of "dagnabbit" reaction. But then miraculously, nightmarishly, he recovered. He seemed now to rear up on his hindquarters in rage. In the next half minute, I emptied half of the can on him; he glistened with the stuff, yet continued to careen into the wall of the bathtub, a dull thud sounding with each impact; it was as if he wanted to dash himself rather than just roll over and die. Finally, though, the chemicals took their toll. He began to list back and forth, and I knew the end was near. He made his way toward me. His last stand. He collected himself and stood motionless once again. There was, in truth, a nobility about him. He was asking for death, not like a beggar, but like an adversary, a noble warrior overcome by superior force. So I gave him the toxic gift. One last squirt, and it was over.

As I opened all the windows to let in fresh air, and to let out the haze of roach spray, another chapter in the struggle between man and the elements in Manhattan had come to an end. And I knew I was a city boy for life.

STUDENT CONFIDENTIAL

It was the second week of the fall semester, the first semester I taught at the Fashion Institute of Technology. It was a Tuesday afternoon, around three o'clock when I boarded the uptown 1 train at Twenty-Eighth Street. The car was crowded, but I lucked out and claimed an end seat when another passenger, realizing at the last instant he was about to miss his stop, jumped up and hopped off the train just as the doors slid shut. I unzipped my backpack for the newspaper inside. But as I pulled out the paper, I made a tactical error—the first, as it turned out, of several.

I looked up.

There, sitting straight across from me, was a pretty young woman with streaming blond hair and a beige tank top. For a moment, I forgot where I was; I forgot that I'd just boarded a train across the street from the college. For a moment, she was only a pretty young woman on a grimy subway car, and I was pleased to be sitting across from her. But that momentary glance proved costly. For she too made the mistake of looking up, and our eyes met in an irrevocable way. She recognized me, and I recognized the fact that she recognized me. I realized, a split second later, that she was my student.

I had no idea what her name was.

"Hi, Professor," she said.

"Hi." Then I improvised: "Heading uptown?"

"Yeah. You?"

"Yeah."

She started to giggle. "Then I guess we both got on the right train."

"I guess so."

What ensued was a silence of perhaps ten seconds, a silence intensified to an unbearable degree because our brief exchange had made us the focal point of our end of the subway car. More than a dozen eavesdroppers in the seats around us were starting to squirm. My eyes scoured the overhead ads for a likely topic of conversation. Abortion hotlines. Hemorrhoid treatment ads. Public health notices. I glanced back at my student. For the first time, I noticed the black binder resting on her lap; it was a modeling portfolio—a familiar sight at the Fashion Institute of Technology.

At least, I figured, the thing would have her name inside.

"Do you model?" I asked.

Instantly, we regained our audience; I felt the tension ease.

She glanced down at the binder. "Just a little bit so far."

"May I see your portfolio?"

As soon as I spoke the words, I wanted to take them back. There was a discernable "uh-oh" in her expression, a sudden sidelong shift of her pupils, followed by a widening of her eyes. Nothing good was going to come of this. But she, too, realized that we had an audience, that her refusal to hand over the portfolio would only draw even more attention to us.

Glancing down, she leaned forward and passed me her portfolio.

Not since I was assigned Henry James's *The Golden Bowl* as a sophomore at Queens College have I less wanted to crack open a book. But I could feel the eyes of a dozen or so onlookers bearing down on me, angling their bodies and craning their necks for a peek; I couldn't very well just sit there with the book on my lap. So I sneaked a final look back across the aisle at my student. She was still staring straight down at the subway floor.

I opened the portfolio and found her name embossed on the inside cover: *Heather.* Across from her name, between plastic flaps, were multiple copies of her one-page résumé. I gave the document a cursory glance, then turned the page.

The first photograph startled me. It was a black and white headshot, with her blond hair pulled up into a tight French braid. What startled me was the feel of the thing, the subtle play of light and shadow. The camera seemed to add not only years but sophistication. The young woman seated across from me couldn't have carried off that expression in person; it would have seemed like playacting, like a little girl trying on her mother's makeup.

To cut the tension, I wanted to ask a professional question. So I mustered up the one relevant term I still recalled from my high school photography class. "I like the *composition* here."

"Yeah," Heather replied. "I think he was good at that."

I nodded at her, then flipped the page.

The second photo was also a headshot, this one in profile. It had the look of an old Greta Garbo promotional still, accentuating the lines of her nose, throat, and cheekbones. Again, it was difficult to imagine that Heather, sitting across from me in faded jeans with both knees torn out, could be photographed to that effect.

I gave the second photo a long look—due diligence, I thought—then, once again, flipped the page.

As soon as I saw the third photo, I understood Heather's reluctance to hand over the portfolio. It was a color image, a full body shot, patterned after a *Cosmo* cover. She was wearing cutoff jean shorts that rode down only an inch or two on her thighs; her plaid work shirt was unbuttoned and tied in a knot high up on her midriff, exposing both her navel and the inside curve of both of her breasts. If I passed it on a newsstand, I wouldn't have given the picture a second glance. From her perspective, however, it wasn't exactly the way you'd want your English professor looking at you.

Again, I thought I'd put her at ease. "The lighting here is very interesting. Do you know what kind of camera the photographer used?"

Heather looked at me with a glimmer of hope but shook her head. Her expression seemed to say: *Why would I know a thing like that?*

Again, I flipped the page.

The third photo was Heather lying nude on a black leather sofa.

The fourth photo was Heather lying nude on a black shag rug.

The fifth photo was Heather standing nude against a black wall.

I wouldn't have gotten to the fourth photo except for the panic I felt at the third; I wouldn't have gotten to the fifth except for the panic I felt at the fourth. But the fifth was as far as I got. After the nanosecond each I spent on photos three, four, and five, I had the presence of mind to slide the portfolio closed.

I heard a young man mutter, "Holy sheeeeeet!"

That elicited giggles from several other riders.

I looked up at Heather. She would not meet my eyes. I shoved the portfolio in her direction, and she took it and held it tightly on her lap. Several seconds later, the train pulled into the station at Times Square. Heather jumped up from her seat and rushed out onto the platform. Whether it was her stop, or she just felt compelled to exit, I did not know.

There was still the minor issue of the rest of the semester for Heather and me. For the next thirteen weeks, we tenaciously avoided eye contact. When I was observed by a senior faculty member, as required by contract, her only quibble with my classroom performance was that I tended to look primarily to the right as I lectured. (Heather sat on the far-left side of the room.) Heather did her assignments each week, did them diligently, revised her work for higher grades as warranted, but she did not say a word in class, and I did not call on her to speak.

That was how I assumed the term would end—with neither of us having mentioned the incident on the train. But during the final exam, I noticed out of the corner of my eye that she was stalling. She'd finished writing her essay, but she had not handed in her blue book. After an hour and a half, she and I were alone in the classroom. Only then did she close her blue book and bring it to the front of the room.

"Professor, I just wanted to say how sorry I was—"

"I'm the one who should be apologizing, Heather."

"The thing is, I got bad advice. I had an agent—"

"You don't owe me an explanation. I should have minded my own business."

"He said I needed to have pictures like that. I did it, but that's not who I am."

I shook my head.

"I have another agent now."

For the first time in thirteen weeks, I looked her in the eyes. "Sounds like the right move."

"It made me re-think what I was doing, what happened on the train. So I guess it turned out okay. It was a good thing you asked to see it. The portfolio, I mean. I'm glad it happened."

As I stared up at her, she began to smile. I realized that she was lying through her teeth—at least about being glad it had happened. She was lying through her teeth for my sake. She wanted me to feel all right about it.

Right there, at that moment, I caught a glimpse of the sophistication from that first black and white head shot. It wasn't in the lighting. It wasn't in the camera angle. It had been in her all along.

THE DOG WALK

When Piper, a friend of mine, asked me to take in Piper, his dachshund, for a weekend, I jumped at the chance. Not that I am a great friend of dogs. But Piper-the-person had gone way into the black on our favor ledger: had watered plants while I was away, had helped me put up a kitchen shelf, had introduced me to his tax guy *etc.* He was at least half a dozen favors up, which was beginning to unnerve me. Moreover, I knew he was desperate, and I knew that in the mathematics of such things one favor can cancel out a half dozen if someone is desperate enough. So I told him he could drop off Piper-the-dog Friday.

Piper-the-person had warned me in advance that Piper-the-dog was old. But the dog he showed up with wasn't just old; he was superannuated, the Methuselah of dogs. The frankfurter body had rounded into knackwurst shape; even his leather leash seemed to droop and drag. It took the dog two tries to hoist his backside across the threshold of my apartment . . . at which point, spent by the effort, he curled up on the cool wood floor and shut his eyes.

"He likes it here," Piper-the-person declared.

"How often should I walk him?"

"Two or three times a day. He'll start to walk in circles near the door." Piper-the-person then handed me a knapsack of dog stuff: cans of soft food, a box of biscuits, a water dish, and a rubber ball stained with dried spit.

"What if he doesn't circle?" I asked.

"Then don't worry. He's independent. He'll let you know what he needs. Dachshunds are very smart dogs, you know. Farmers use them to hunt badgers. They follow the badgers underground, and the badgers try to trick them into false burrows and bury them alive. They learn to think for themselves."

The Pipers then exchanged their goodbyes, and moments later Piper-the-person was gone.

I patted the dog on the head. "Just you and me, boy."

He shut his eyes again.

For the next forty-eight hours, Piper-the-dog was an ideal guest. He sucked down his meals, lapped his water dish dry, did his circle dance at regular intervals. Mostly, though, he just lay around, a cross between an ottoman and a throw rug. Every now and then, I would glance over at him and mutter, "Easy there, boy." By Sunday evening, as I took him downstairs, I'd grown fond of him; I even felt a twinge at the thought that he would be gone the following morning.

As usual, after three minutes, the business end of our walk was done. I decided, because it was our last night, to take him once around the block—a twenty-minute trek at Piper's pace, but the night breeze was warm, and the sky was cloudless. So off we went. I paid little attention to him, allowed him to walk me, my thoughts wandering up toward a perfect crescent moon.

Several minutes later, I felt a tug on the leash. Piper had nosed his way into a pile of newspapers beside the curb. I gave the leash a pull, but the dog dug in his heels; he would not be moved. I pulled harder, to no avail. He'd found something. His entire body had stiffened with the effort to take hold of it. Finally, I leaned over for a better look.

He had a dead pigeon in his mouth.

Now, in an instant, Piper was transformed: The badger dog of his youth returned. He sensed prey in his jaws. Triumphant, he met my eyes—and then, with a sudden burst that almost yanked my arm from its socket, he dashed for home, for my apartment. He was a low-flying missile as I stumbled after him. It took me perhaps seven steps to regain my balance, to plant my feet and drag him to a halt. The leash was like a tightrope between us. I could hear low growls issue from the innermost recesses of his being; I had to gather the leash with both hands to get at him, to climb down to his collar. When I finally collared him, I saw that he had the pigeon full in his mouth, two twig-like legs visible between his teeth . . . there was no question that he was about to ingest the bird. This struck me as a bad outcome. If he'd caught the thing and killed it himself, maybe; but this pigeon had died of pigeon disease. Given Piper's age, I didn't like the odds of his surviving such a meal.

I had to get the pigeon out of his mouth.

Life, unfortunately, had not prepared me for this moment. As I grabbed what I could of the pigeon's body, the growling started again. This was his prize, his triumph, and I was trying to rob him of it. "C'mon boy," I whispered, "let go." He braced his legs against the sidewalk. It was a standoff; I had enough of the bird in my grasp to stop him from chewing it but not enough to take it from him. For a minute, Piper and I stared each other down.

Then, at last, I heard a voice behind me. "Hey, man, you got to get that away from him." It was Florian, the guy who operated the corner kiosk.

"I'm trying," I managed.

"He eats that, forget about it!"

Florian knelt down beside me and tried to force open Piper's jaws with his fingers. The dog shook his head from side to side but wouldn't let go. Then Florian nudged my hands aside and laid hold of the bird himself; he took it and lifted Piper three feet off the ground. Still, the dog would not give up his grip. I sat on the sidewalk and watched in astonishment. It looked like a circus act.

"Tickle his stomach," Florian said.

This I did—although I had no clue why. Then at once I heard a tearing sound, and then another; feathers began fluttering to the ground all around me. When I glanced up, Florian was flinging pigeon parts, recognizable pigeon parts, wings and legs, into the gutter. Piper started to bark in dismay and tumbled to earth an instant later. Except for a few feathers, his mouth was clear.

When I looked up to thank Florian, he'd already started to wander off. He called back, "No problem, man." Then I glanced down at Piper-the-dog. The years had returned to him; the sag was back. He coughed up the last of the feathers, and we began the slow walk home.

CROTCH KILLER

If I had an American Indian nickname, it would be Crotch Killer. The muscles in my thighs are squared off and thick—the physiological signature of a former sprinter—and rub together as I walk. That friction, in turn, causes me to wear out pants the same way time after time.

Right below the crotch.

The process starts the first time I slide on a new pair of pants. Within the first few hundred steps, the material between the upper thighs has begun to fray. By the third time through the wash, the material has become translucent. By the sixth time or seventh time, there is a fissure. By the eighth time, the pants have become unwearable . . . though they still look fine everywhere but the crotch.

Jeans last significantly longer because the material is tougher, but the outcome is still the same. With jeans, however, I often adopt an I-meant-to-wear-them-like-that attitude even once the telltale breeze rears up from below. I feel justified in this by racks of pre-torn designer brands found in posh boutiques. If shredded knees count as the height of fashion, why should a hidden breach of the inner sanctum disqualify otherwise comfortable pants?

Still, I am always on the lookout for another pair. Pants, I confess, intrigue me in ways no other garments do. For one thing, there's the issue of sizing. I'm five feet, nine inches tall, roughly the planetary average for male Homo sapiens. I weigh one sixty-five most of the time, which also puts me within one standard deviation of the norm among well-fed Americans. What that translates into, as far as pants are concerned, is a thirty-inch inseam and a thirty-three-inch waist. The latter is occasionally problematic; many brand-name companies only manufacture even-numbered waists. But a thirty-four cinches up awkwardly as soon as I pull a belt around it, and the backside hangs off my butt as though I've got a full diaper underneath. On the other hand, a thirty-two forces me to go long periods without exhaling, and the pant legs gather around my thighs like sausage skins. What is the possible rationale for a clothing company to exclude odd-numbered waistlines from their men's catalogues? This strikes me as a civil rights issue. I hope there's litigation pending.

Even more puzzling than waists are inseams. As I said, I'm just about the median height for planet Earth and have a thirty-inch inseam. But inseam sizes seem to *start* at thirty inches. I don't think I've ever seen a twenty-nine on a department store rack. If half the world's males are shorter than I am, where do they shop? These, I think, must be the Great Hemming Masses—men who never get to wear new pants off the rack, in their pristine retail state, and who must therefore factor the cost of alterations into the purchase price. To put the matter in perspective: I've seen a twenty-eight-inch waist with a forty-two-inch inseam hanging in an upscale Fifth Avenue shop . . . just in case Dennis Rodman happens to wander in. (Though in that case shouldn't it be in the woman's section?) But I've never seen the reverse, a forty-two/twenty-eight, which would fit about half the tourists at the Times Square Applebee's.

Pants styles come and go without rhyme or reason. Occasionally, I can get behind one. Pleats, for example, during their Kid Creole and the Coconuts heyday in the 1980s, were a welcome relief on the thigh level. But pleated fabrics were often so delicate that the first whisper of contact between my legs burned through them like a blowtorch. I was never a fan of bell-bottoms—too many memories of that grotesque

Keep on Truckin' poster from the late sixties. (Though I do recall that bell-bottoms were much easier to pull off and on over sneakers in high school gym class.) Button flies are a Luddite nuisance; the invention of the zipper was a technological advance, a genuine leap forward in civilization, so what's the point of going back? Oh, and I'd like to meet the genius who came up with idea of "dirty denim" . . . *yeah, these should go great with my stepped-in-crap Hush Puppies.*

Then there's the distinction between chinos and khakis. Many people whom I trust tell me that there is one, but I cannot grasp it. They explain that chinos are dressier than khakis, even though chinos can be khaki in color, and that chinos are twilled cotton, but khakis can be either twilled or not twilled, and sometimes not cotton but linen, even though linen itself can be made out of cotton. My eyes tend to glaze over at this point as the entire issue takes the form of an LSAT question.

Currently, I own eighteen pairs of pants. I rarely ever wear fourteen of them; either they've gone out of style, or never were in style, or seemed like a good idea at the time I bought them but proved otherwise—for example, a pair of white jeans I picked up after a friend invited me out on his boat, only to find that the glare off the pants blinded him as he steered along the Hudson River. I don't wear three of the other pairs of pants because their tags say "dry clean only"—which, in Manhattan, means getting taken to the cleaners in quite another sense.

The greatest pants I ever owned were a pair of slate gray Perry Ellis dress slacks. The material, as I recall, was a synthetic of polyester, baby's bottom, and a Miles Davis trumpet solo; putting them on felt like sliding into shaving cream lather. They hugged without binding, flowed without billowing. According to their care label, they were "machine washable/wrinkle resistant," but that understated the point. Those guys came out of the washer looking *improved* each time.

Except, of course, where it counted most. It was heart-wrenching to watch them disintegrate at the critical juncture. I lived in sartorial denial, didn't wear them for several months with the thought that somehow, with rest, the pants would heal, that they would recover the splendid vigor of their youth. But it wasn't to be. They were undone by a force greater than mere warp and woof.

They were undone by Crotch Killer.

THE BASEBALL CARD

According to a recent price guide, five dollars will get you a mint-condition 1967 baseball card with two New York Yankees rookies, Stan Bahnsen and Bobby Murcer. That's roughly one percent of the going rate for a mint-condition 1968 Jerry Koosman-Nolan Ryan rookie card. Cash value and emotional value of course are distinct measures. I idolized Bobby Murcer in the late 1960s, and his rookie card was, during the brief time I owned it, the most cherished possession of my childhood.

How did Bobby Murcer become my favorite baseball player? He was a Yankee, so he had the definite advantage of showing up on local TV. I also remember looking at the 1967 rookie card and liking his face—so round and lit up by a smile that his teammates would later nickname him "Lemon." Then, too, there was the name Bobby. Bobby Richardson, the Yankees' longtime second baseman, had been the first ballplayer I followed, and he'd just retired, so I was in the market for a new favorite. Plus, Murcer was a *true* Bobby. That was his actual first name. Not Robert. Not Rob. Not Bob. I mean, Bobby was something you were *called*, not something you were *named*. Bobby Richardson was Robert Clinton Richardson. Bobby Kennedy was Robert Francis

Kennedy. But Bobby Murcer was Bobby Ray Murcer. No Robert about it. That sealed the deal.

Murcer got called up to the big leagues for the proverbial cup of coffee in '66 and '67, then served in the army for two years—which struck me as exceptionally brave, so I remained true to him even though he was gone until 1969. By the time he returned to the majors, my devotion to him was absolute. I was eleven at the start of that season, and I began reading the newspapers my father brought home in order to track his statistics; I jumped to the head of my class in fractions and decimals by calculating his batting average day by day.

When Murcer was hitting, life was good. Existential concerns were not to forget my clip-on tie on assembly Thursdays and not to flinch when I got my booster shots. Those were halcyon days of gender-specific toys, of Dolly Darlings and Matchbox Racers, and of relatives who could be counted on to reinforce societal stereotypes. Thanksgivings were to be endured because aunts and uncles arrived with ten-packs of Topps baseball cards . . . always the old series, to be sure, but even these were useful to scale during recess and as trade bait whenever a teacher left the room. Such were the pre-lapsarian days of card collecting, when the notion of resale would have been laughable, indeed incomprehensible, when "got it" and "need it" were the main determinants of free-market worth, and when every boy on the block had his own checklist of untouchables—cards too dear ever to part with.

My checklist of untouchables—apart from Bobby Murcer, who in truth belonged to a separate category—included Johnny Callison, Jerry Koosman, Willie Davis, and Jim Lefebvre. (I'm struck, in retrospect, by the fact that none of them is a Hall of Famer; with the exception of Murcer, who starred on a handful of miserable Yankees teams in the late 1960s and early 1970s, each was probably the second-best player on his team. While the rest of my friends were idolizing Aaron and Mays and Banks and Seaver and Clemente, I gathered the near-greats closest to my breast.) These were the cards I kept tucked away in my sock-and-underwear drawer. My Bobby Murcer rookie card, on the other hand, sat upright on my desk, leaning against the base of my tensor lamp, where I could keep an eye on it as I did my homework.

It was the onset of puberty, that source of unending mischief and chagrin, that cost me Bobby Murcer. In a moment of weakness, I gave the card to Heidi Rifkin, the first girl I ever got to like me. To consecrate our eternal union, she insisted we exchange our most precious possessions. Heidi gave me her forty-five-rpm single of Bobby Sherman singing "Little Woman." I forked over Bobby Murcer. It was the sort of gesture that only the idiotic sincerity of a thirteen-year-old boy can produce; had I handed her Bobby Knoop, she would've never known the difference. And when we broke up less than a month later, Heidi flung the card back in my face. In two pieces. (Her Bobby Sherman record, I might add, was returned without a scratch.) She had sheared the card in half, straight down the middle; she'd severed Bahnsen from Murcer. The cut was precise, surgical—a metaphor, in a way, for any number of future involvements with women. Scotch tape does no good in such situations. I didn't even keep the halves.

That would be the end of the story, and a rather sad one, except that I awakened on my thirty-fifth birthday with a sudden, throbbing need to reacquire a 1967 Bobby Murcer rookie card. Now this was in June 1992, long before Google and eBay, so for that entire summer I became a knight errant, and a baseball card my holy grail, and I would prowl the folding card tables along Fifth Avenue, my fingers crossed, standing patiently in the warm breeze as an eighteen-year-old hustler tried to pawn off a 3-D Deion Sanders—which, he swore, would quadruple in value within a decade. He and his pimply-faced competitors would expound on the relative merits of various brands of cards, of Fleer and Donruss, of Score and Upper Deck. (The Topps monopoly was by then long gone.) Their tables were stacked with basketball and football cards, with Star Trek and Desert Storm cards, with cards of pro wrestlers and of Elvis, cards of The Little Mermaid and of Harley-Davidson motorcycles. There were also special adults-only series with names like "the Centerfold Collection" and "California Girls." Another set that caught my eye was called "Crime and Punishment," which had nothing to do with Dostoevsky; its lineup included Charles Manson, Ted Bundy, and Jeffrey Dahmer. "It was banned in a lot of states," the sales-kid said, with an air of theatrical confidentiality. "It's gonna be worth *beaucoup* bucks in a couple of years, you mark my words."

I walked on.

As summer wound into fall, and then fall into winter, and the card tables on Fifth Avenue folded up shop, I began journeying to the outer boroughs, deep into the bowels of Brooklyn and Queens, and once even to Long Island, to attend card shows. These were dispiriting events, put together by jowly middle-aged dealers sporting gray-flecked ponytails and protruding guts that hung several inches below the hem of their heavy-metal tee shirts. Many of them, it turned out, still lived in their parents' houses—in the basement, they were quick to add . . . *so, really, if you stop and think about it, it's the same thing as having your own place, except you don't have to do laundry, so you tell me who's the real schmuck?* Several claimed to have a Murcer rookie card, except not with them, but if I joined their mailing list, they'd be sure to bring the card to the next show (which always seemed to be in New Jersey). I was tempted. But many years before, I'd signed up for an evangelical mailing list—because I wanted a Bible concordance, and I got one for free if I signed up—and those people hounded me for over a decade, across three moves and a half dozen return-to-sender notes, until at last a lawyer friend lent me a sheet of his firm's stationery, and I wrote them a bluff cease-and-desist letter. That did the trick.

The start of baseball season the next spring quickened my desperation to find a Bobby Murcer rookie card. Murcer, at that time, was a TV broadcaster for the Yankees, so the sound of his voice every night was like a drumbeat of want. Near the end of April, I devised a new plan. I'd embarked on a second career as a newspaper columnist, and I was writing semi-regular columns for *Newsday*. Surely in the attic of one of my readers lay a Bobby Murcer rookie card collecting dust! That was the parlay I had in mind when I published a piece called "Bobby Murcer is my Dulcinea" on May 20, 1993. (You could look it up!) In the column, I detailed the grievous wrong done to me by Heidi Rifkin, and my determination to replace the Bobby Murcer rookie card. (The column's title, I should add, wasn't my idea: "Dulcinea" is the lady-love of the title character in *Don Quixote* by Cervantes; she appears nowhere in the actual book, but we learn that Don Quixote idealizes and idolizes her, and that her flesh-and-blood counterpart, Aldonza Lorenzo, as described by Sancho Panza, is, shall we say, somewhat earthier. By contrast, my quest for the Murcer card, if it had a precursor among literary romances, was more like Dante's quest to return to the innocent perfection of his youthful love for Beatrice.)

Two days after the column appeared, I got a call from a guy in Dobbs Ferry. He'd read my column in *Newsday* and found my number in the telephone book, and, sure enough, he had (in his attic!) a mint-condition 1967 Bobby Murcer rookie card . . . which he was willing to trade for the original manuscript of the newspaper column. Was I interested?

"You bet," I said.

So I printed out another hard copy of the column—I had no idea what the editors at *Newsday* had done with the original—made a few markings in red ink so that it looked authentic, and the next morning hopped a Metro North train out of Grand Central for the half-hour ride to Dobbs Ferry. We made the exchange in the guy's driveway. He examined the six typed pages, and I stared in rapture at the baseball card. Then we shook hands and parted. Just like that, I had a 1967 Bobby Murcer rookie card.

On the ride back to Manhattan, I was reveling not only in the fact that I once again owned the object I'd devoted a year of my life to tracking down, but also that I'd bent reality to my will. I'd devised a plan to get the thing, and by gum the plan had worked. The result was tangible. I was sitting on a Metro North train, holding the card in my right hand.

I was still holding it in my right hand when I got back to my Midtown apartment. I brought it over to my desk, leaned it against the base of my halogen lamp, and for several minutes I sat there and revered it. Then, out of the corner of my eye, I noticed the blinking red light on my answering machine. I had a message. Reluctantly, I got up from the desk and pressed the button on the machine: "Hey, I hope this is the Mark Goldblatt who writes for *Newsday*. My name is John Moore. I direct the Yankee broadcasts on WPIX. I wanted to let you know that Bobby got a real kick out of your article the other day, and he'd like to meet you. How'd you feel about coming down to the stadium this week and joining us for an inning in the booth?"

I called the number he left and said, "You bet."

Which was how I wound up at Yankee Stadium on Tuesday evening, May 25, 1993. As I rode the escalator to the press level, escorted by a security guard, I remember thinking that maybe I'd done more than bend reality to my will; maybe I'd warped reality altogether—since under no plausible circumstances were my life and Bobby Murcer's life supposed to intersect. Yet a minute later I was standing at the curtained entrance of the Yankees broadcast booth, and the security guard was patting me on the back and telling me to go inside.

The first guy to greet me on the other side of the curtain was John Moore. He was younger than I'd imagined him, maybe my age, with a shock of light brown hair and the generic facial features of a dairy farmer. He shook my hand and told me how much he'd liked my *Newsday* column. Then he said, "Let me introduce you to the guys."

The *guys* were Phil Rizzuto, Tom Seaver . . . and Bobby Murcer.

The three of them were sitting in the front of the booth with their backs to me, prepping for the game against the Orioles.

"Hey, Phil," John Moore called, "I got someone I'd like you to meet."

Rizzuto turned around and got out of his chair. He hopped up the three long steps to the back of the booth, a tight bundle of nervous energy. "You Goldberg?"

I nodded: If Phil Rizzuto thought I was Goldberg, who was I to argue?

He shook my hand, then said, "Hey, loved your article. You're a Murcer fan, eh? What do you know! Let me introduce you . . ."

I didn't hear much after that. I followed Rizzuto back down the three steps to the front of the booth, where Tom Seaver and Bobby Murcer were sitting. Seaver was the first to look up. We made eye contact, and I put out my hand; he shook it, reluctantly. I could tell by the look on his face that he had no idea who I was, or what I was doing in the broadcast booth, and he didn't seem pleased that I was there, so I didn't try to explain things. I just mumbled a quick hello and moved on.

Bobby Murcer still hadn't looked up. He was wearing a set of black headphones, listening to a voice that I could hear but not quite make out. He didn't realize Rizzuto and I were standing behind him until Rizzuto leaned forward and tapped him on the shoulder. He glanced back, smiled his 1967 rookie card smile, then pulled off the headphones and stood up.

I shook hands with Bobby Murcer.

"Well hello there, young man!" he said, in a thick Southern drawl. (It's good to keep in mind that I was thirty-five years old, and Murcer had just turned forty-seven.) It occurred to me, as I held on to his hand for a split second too long, that he was probably more accustomed to shaking hands with kids going through chemotherapy than with the likes of me. "I read your article, and I'm mighty glad to know you."

I finally let go of his hand. "I'm honored.... I'm just so... honored. It's an honor."

"I'm sure you hear this all the time, but you've got a real way with words."

"Big words!" Rizzuto added.

"Yeah, *real* big words," Murcer said. "We were kind of laughing about that, how you must've memorized the entire dictionary."

"Nah..."

"What was that word we were talking about, Scooter?"

Rizzuto said, "Oh, *that* one... it was pre-*something*."

"*Prelapsarian*?" I said.

"Yeah, that's it. We couldn't even *find* that one."

"It means before the Fall," I said.

"Yeah?"

"Before Adam and Eve ate the—"

"The apple?" Rizzuto said.

"Well, actually, it's the fruit of the tree of the knowledge of good and evil—"

"How do you like that, Murcer? I always thought it was an apple! Live and learn. What was that other word? *Existential?*"

"That just means what actually exists," I said. "You know, in the here and now."

"I told you so!" Rizzuto shouted.

"There's a whole school of philosophy called existentialism—"

Rizzuto took a step back. "Whoa, this conversation's getting too deep for me. I'll leave the two of you alone."

Murcer stepped forward at that point and put his arm around my shoulder. "You teach at a fashion school, right?"

Oh great . . . my childhood idol thinks I'm gay . . . there's not even a name for that complex . . .

"It's a branch of the state university . . ."

"Where'd you learn so many big words?"

"I guess I just picked them up through the years."

"Did you play baseball growing up?" he asked.

"Softball more than baseball. I still play in a couple of leagues."

"What position?"

"Right center field," I said.

"*Right* center field?"

"There are four outfielders in softball."

"Oh, yeah, that's right," he said.

There followed an awkward silence.

Then Murcer said, "So I hear you're going to call a half inning with us."

"I am?"

"That's what Moore told me." He scanned the booth and located John Moore at the rear, reading over a clipboard of notes. "Hey, John! My buddy Mark's going to call a half inning, right?"

John Moore flashed him a thumbs-up.

"Which one?" Murcer asked.

"Home, third," Moore called back.

Murcer looked me straight in the eyes. "You nervous?"

"Not until right now," I said.

"We'll just ask you a few questions about your article. It'll go pretty fast."

"What if there's a rally?"

He laughed. "Then just keep talking."

With that, he turned and walked back to his broadcast position, and I took a seat in the rear of the booth, next to John Moore.

The game started a couple of minutes later, and the first two and a half innings were unremarkable. As the bottom of the third approached, Moore leaned over to me and whispered, "Nervous?"

"Only when someone asks me if I'm nervous."

"The big thing you have to remember is don't talk when the ball's in play."

"That seems pretty easy to remember," I said.

"Tell it to Rizzuto!"

Half a minute later, during an extended commercial, Moore nudged me, and I walked down to the front of the booth. With a last look of disdain, Seaver stood up and gave me his chair then headed out for a coffee break. Murcer picked up Seaver's abandoned headset and handed it to me, and I sat down. The moment I put on the headset, nerves kicked in . . . I was about to be on television in front of a million people. *Literally, a million people.* My neck stiffened to an iron rod, and my stomach dissolved to jelly. There was a thirteen-inch monitor in front of me; the screen flickered for a split second, and then an image came up of Rizzuto, Murcer, and me taken from the center-field camera—well over a hundred yards away. Even at that distance, my eyes were the size of grapes. I was identified by white letters superimposed across my chest: "Mark Goldblatt. Newsday Columnist. Murcer Fan."

The commercial ended, a red light on the monitor went on, and we were on the air.

Rizzuto began, "We've got a special guest in the booth today. It's Mark Goldblatt. Did I get that right?"

I nodded. Just nodded.

"So anyway, Mark's a columnist for *Newsday*, and he's also a Murcer fan. Isn't that right?"

I nodded again, vigorously.

My neck began to pulse.

"You want to tell your story, Mark?" Rizzuto said.

My voice cracked as I started to speak: "Well, you see, the thing is, Bobby Murcer was always my favorite ballplayer when I was growing up, and his 1967 rookie card was my prize possession, and when I was twelve, I gave it to a girl I liked—"

"Okay, we'll get back to that in a minute. We got Mike Gallego stepping to the plate against Jamie Moyer . . ."

I took deep breaths as Rizzuto and Murcer called Mike Gallego's at bat. I was half hoping they'd forget about me, but the moment Gallego grounded out to third base, the center-field camera again zoomed in on the three of us in the broadcast booth. Rizzuto swiveled his chair sideways and said, "So, Mark, you were talking about that Bobby Murcer rookie card . . ."

"Yeah, well, I gave it to this girl in my sixth-grade class, and then, after we parted ways, she cut the card in half—"

"Ouch!" Murcer chimed in.

"Yeah, it was a clean cut, right down the middle," I said. "Stan Bahnsen went one way, and you went the other. I didn't think about it much for, like, twenty years, but then, last year, I woke up one morning, and I wanted that card back. So I started to travel to card shows in Brooklyn and Long Island—"

"All right, we got Wade Boggs digging in against Moyer . . ."

Boggs lined a single to left, made a wide turn at first base, but trotted back to the bag. Once that bit of business was over, the center-field camera zoomed back in on the booth.

Rizzuto said, "So in the end did you get the card back or not?"

"Well, yeah, I did," I said. "Just a few days ago, as a matter of fact, after *Newsday* published my column—"

"You hear that, Murcer? Sounds like this guy went to a lot of trouble to get your card back."

"He sure did, Scooter, and don't think I don't appreciate it."

"All right," Rizzuto said, "we got Jim Leyritz coming to bat against Jamie Moyer with a runner on first and one out . . ."

I took a deep breath. I assumed the interview was over, and I started to get up, but Murcer put his hand and held up a sheet of paper. On it, he'd written the words, "You call the next play."

I mouthed the word, "Me?"

He nodded; I glanced over at Rizzuto, who was also nodding.

Right then, Moyer threw a pitch and Leyritz swung.

For a half second, there was only silence. Dead air.

Then I said, "Leyritz hits a weak ground ball to the first baseman, who tosses to second for the force play."

"Hey, nice job, buddy!" Murcer said, on air.

"Way to go!" Rizzuto added. "You're a natural."

"I don't even know the first baseman's name."

"You think I do?" Rizzuto said.

The three of us laughed. *On air*. Suddenly, I was one of the guys. I felt a wave of confidence wash over me. I said, "All right, now it's Mike Stanley's turn to see what he can do against Jamie Moyer . . ."

Murcer gave me an encouraging shove as Stanley stepped into the batter's box.

"So, Bobby," I said, "do you know what I've always wondered?"

"What's that?"

"The runner on first base, he's got like a ten-foot lead, right?"

"Yeah?"

"But he can get picked off, right?"

"That's the deal," Murcer said.

"Don't you think he'd get a quicker start if he gave up the ten-foot lead, got into a sprinter's stance, and used the first-base bag as a starting block?"

Dead silence.

"Plus," I said, "he wouldn't have to worry about getting picked off. I realize he'd have to run an extra ten feet to steal second base, but I think he'd still get there faster if he pushed off the first-base bag—I mean, that's why Olympic sprinters use starting blocks."

Murcer started to laugh. "Friend, that might work in *softball*, but this is Major League Baseball . . ."

Then Rizzuto said, "Swing and a miss. Strike one on Mike Stanley."

Just like that, it was over. I felt John Moore tap me on the shoulder, and I heard Rizzuto say, "We're going to have to say goodbye to our friend Mark, who got his Bobby Murcer card. So there's a happy ending for you. Now let's see if the Yankees can manage a happy ending tonight against the O's."

Murcer gave my shoulder one last squeeze as I set down the headset.

For the record, the Yankees won the game one to nothing. Winning pitcher: Bob Wickman. Losing pitcher: Jamie Moyer.

When I got home, I had twenty-seven messages on my answering machine. Or twenty-four more than I'd ever had before. My softball coach asked me why I'd pissed off Murcer with the leading-off thing. (I told him I hadn't.) My dissertation advisor told me how proud he was to be working with me. (My dissertation itself had no similar effect.) My mother told me not to get a big head. (Too late, by a couple of decades.)

Oh, I *still* think a runner would get to second base faster out of a sprinter's stance . . .

THE QUESTIONNAIRE

It was through softball in Central Park that I met Annie, the woman who would introduce me to the world of online dating. There is a great deal to admire about her, not the least of which is the fact that she broke the gender barrier in our Sunday-morning softball league. She is entrenched as the starting pitcher of the Viaducts—once a ragtag outfit of lovable losers but now, since Annie joined them, a perennial playoff contender and onetime league champion. The Viaducts used to be called Mild Head Injury, but Annie urged them to change their name; she made it a condition of her signing on. If you come to the field expecting to lose and thinking your team is a joke, she said, you *will* lose and your team *will* be a joke. So Mild Head Injury became the Viaducts—a bastardization of *Ducts*, which is the name of a literary webzine founded by the team's center fielder and captain, Jonathan.

Annie also lobbied for a change of uniforms from their traditional gray pullovers to button-down pastel blue jerseys, with the Viaducts logo—which she designed herself—emblazoned across the chest. Style counts when you're putting together a winning tradition. So does physical presence . . . and Annie is an absolute sight on the mound, six feet tall and put together like a Radio City Rockette, taking one giant stride toward home plate before she releases the ball. She throws a deceptive riser and mixes in an occasional straight change, but perhaps the most unnerving aspect of batting against her is the knowledge that she inscribes the name of every hitter she strikes out on the underside brim of her cap.

My name is there.

Annie, in sum, is not someone to be taken lightly. So when she suggested that I sign up for eHarmony, I didn't blow off the suggestion. I didn't quite embrace it either. Why would I use the Internet to find dates? After all, I met lots of women through work and at literary events . . .

True, I didn't date any of them. But I met them.

Neither blowing off nor quite embracing Annie's suggestion, I began to canvass friends and acquaintances. They seemed roughly split on the idea. One woman, whom I'd known since junior high school, insisted that the entire phenomenon of dating online was stupid and unnatural. But she went to holistic healers and ate kelp and considered things like modern refrigeration unnatural. On the other side, a lawyer pal of mine told me he'd been doing online dating for three years, juggling several different sites, and had gotten laid more often than kitchen linoleum.

The decisive argument came from my friend Charles, a keen observer of human nature, who had also seen me take a called third strike against Annie. "If you walk into a bar," Charles said, "you're what . . . an epsilon male? Maybe a delta at best? But online you're disembodied. You know lots of words. Your grammar is strong. Online, you might jump straight to alpha."

That cinched it for me.

I glanced at the eHarmony website that night. I was struck at once by the fact that in order to join, I had to answer five hundred questions. Literally, five hundred questions . . . a veritable colonic of the innermost creedal me. It was the brainchild of a family of grinning evangelicals who'd hired a team of "relationship experts" to design the survey. (I Googled the outfit first as a precaution.) Before the grinning evangelicals down at corporate headquarters in Santa Monica, California, would even take my credit card number, they wanted to know more about me than I'd ever confided in another human being. They asked me questions I expected: How often did I drink? (Never.) How often did I smoke? (Never.) How often did I lose my temper? (Never, damn it!) But also questions that caught me off-guard: What did I value more, respect or money? (There was no third option, no space for commentary, no opportunity to point out that money buys respect, so I chose respect because I didn't want to highlight my Jewish ancestry.) How would I assess my verbal intimacy skills? (Luckily, multiple-choice answers were provided.) It was one o'clock in the morning when I reached question 175, which inquired whether or not I considered myself ambitious. As I clicked *no*, I seemed to recall being asked that question, worded in a slightly different way, at least twice before; actually, I was *certain* I'd been asked that question at least three times. I figured the redundancy must be a programming glitch, or maybe human error. But then, a minute later, I realized that the questionnaire was not merely a questionnaire; it was a *test*.

The grinning evangelicals wanted to know if I was lying.

The gauntlet had been thrown, so I pressed on. Past question 250, the halfway point: Did I want children? (Maybe.) There was no turning back now. Even if I never joined, I'd finish the damn survey. I would prove to them that I was eHarmony material. If there's one thing I've learned from years of opinion-column writing, it's that you don't want grinning evangelicals thinking poorly of you.

Question 400: How much significance did I attach to a woman's looks?

Well, of course, I was more interested in what a woman had going on *inside*, in the strength of her character, in her spiritual life, in her . . . oh, who was I kidding? I attached a lot of significance to a woman's looks. That's right, a lot! There, I said it! I want to date Brigitte Bardot! Well, no, she'd be about a hundred years old by now. So maybe her granddaughter. Yeah, I want to date Brigitte Bardot's granddaughter! Do you hear that, Elmer Gantry? Looks matter! Just pull the moving van around the back of my house, and unload the ten finalists for Miss Bible Belt . . .

I went to the kitchen and made myself a cup of coffee.

It was just after three in the morning when I answered question 500: How far was I willing to travel to meet the woman of my dreams? I was determined to select, "I'll travel to the ends of the earth if necessary." But the choices were prosaic, and I lived in Manhattan, and, well, *I lived in Manhattan*, so I clicked "ten miles."

Then, at once, the computer screen shifted. The text of the survey was gone. My data was being processed. Then, after half a minute, another screen came up. I was asked to enter the number and expiration date of my credit card.

Suddenly, as with the flick of a switch, I was lucid again: No way was I going to join eHarmony!

I woke up the next morning with a splitting headache—par for the course, since I'd overslept. I staggered to the bathroom and swallowed a couple of aspirins and another couple of ibuprofens. Then, listlessly, I headed for the computer and discovered that I had three new e-mails. The first came from a Nigerian woman asking me to invest in her late husband's diamond mine. The second came from an Internet drug site that offered discounts on Viagra.

The third came from the grinning evangelicals at eHarmony. It began with an italicized message: *Dear Mark, there's a very special person we'd like you to meet . . .*

That special person was "Pamela from Secaucus, New Jersey."

I followed the link at the bottom of the e-mail back to the eHarmony website—only to be informed that in order to view a photograph or to communicate with Pamela from Secaucus, I had to become a paid member.

For several minutes, I sat at the computer, agonizing over whether to type my credit card number into the eHarmony database. But at last I took the fateful step. I felt a strong sense of dread as I began to type in the card number. After I was done, I pressed the Enter key and held my breath.

Several moments later, the face of Pamela from Secaucus materialized next to her name. She was a pretty blond, in the way of an aging real estate agent, with slightly too much makeup and slightly too wide a smile. I was smitten with her at once. She seemed a fellow traveler, a child of my generation, wearied perhaps but not quite defeated by the circumstances of her life. According to her profile, which now appeared in a long rectangular box below her name and photo, she was a psychotherapist, had been married and divorced; had no children but might want them in the future; considered her mentally challenged younger sister the most influential person in her life; could not live without her iPod, her cell phone, Pepperidge Farm Milano cookies, her family and friends, and love. She didn't smoke, drank only socially, identified herself as "spiritual but not religious," spent her leisure time traveling abroad, listening to classical music, taking long walks and reading "fiction novels." She claimed that the first thing people noticed about her was her laugh and that the one thing people never seemed to notice about her was her sense of humor—which struck me as paradoxical, though not necessarily untrue. The last book she'd read was a Harry Potter fiction novel. Asked to describe one thing about herself that only her best friend would know, she replied, coquettishly, "You'll have to become my best friend and find out for yourself."

I came to the end of her profile, to a tab that read "Click here to begin communication with Pamela from Secaucus."

No trout ever chomped a hook as readily.

The instant I clicked the tab, however, I was confronted with a final set of inquiries; before I could begin communication with Pamela from Secaucus, I had to complete a profile page of my own. Much of the data had been gleaned from the initial barrage of five hundred questions: I worked as a college professor and writer, had never been married, had no children but might want them, did not smoke or drink. But now I was asked more expansive questions: *Whom, not counting my parents, did I consider the most influential person in my life?* I thought at first of Socrates—except there's that nagging man-boy love thing, so I nixed the entire category of Greek philosophers. Next I considered Dostoevsky, and actually typed in D-o-s-t-o, but then, on second thought, backspaced; his marital life was a wreck, he gambled compulsively, and the idea that he was intermittently God-drunk might not sit well with a spiritual-but-not-religious gal like Pamela from Secaucus. The more I thought about the question, the more I came to appreciate her response. To name her handicapped younger sister as the most influential person in her life was a stroke of genius.

It said much about her sense of familial loyalty, about her perspective on life, about the psychotherapeutic kindness of her heart. Could I ask for more in the future Mrs. Mark Goldblatt?

How foolish to have considered Socrates or Dostoevsky! Anonymity was the way to go. So I wrote: "The most influential person in my life, not counting my parents, was a philosophy professor I had in college. He taught me the value of rational arguments, of understanding the moral responsibilities people bear toward one another, and of following the truth in whatever direction it leads. Either him, or David Hasselhoff." That last touch, I felt, was necessary to offset the possible perception of haughtiness. Which is to take nothing away from Mr. Hasselhoff, who I understand is a big man in Germany, one of the few whose résumé does not include crimes against humanity—a debatable point if you've ever heard him sing. But I cannot claim that he's influenced me in any discernable way.

Next, I was asked how I spent my leisure time. To which I responded: 1) Reading. 2) Playing softball. 3) Taking long walks in the city. 4) Answering questions from eHarmony. Then I was asked what people first noticed about me. To which I responded: "The fact that I don't go out of my way to be noticed." Then I was asked what people *don't* notice about me that I wished they would. To which I responded: "The fact that I don't go out of my way to be noticed is actually a desperate cry for attention." Then I was asked to name six things I couldn't live without. To which I responded: 1) Six or more hours of sleep. 2) My laptop computer. 3) C-SPAN. 4) Softball in Central Park. 5) Gravity. 6) *The Norton Anthology of English Literature, Volume One.* Then I was asked the last book I'd read. To which I responded: *The Norton Anthology of English Literature, Volume One.* Then I was asked to describe one thing about me that only my best friend would know. To which I replied: "Only my best friend would know that I just read *The Norton Anthology of English Literature, Volume One* . . . and I've sworn him to secrecy."

Finally, I was asked (though not required) to upload a photo . . . or three. This I did.

I read through the answers one last time, took one last glance at the photos, and pressed Enter. The cheerful message returned, and this time for good: "Click here to begin communication with Pamela from Secaucus."

I clicked.

Here is the first message I sent to Pamela from Secaucus: "I'm new to this and not sure how to proceed, but I wanted to say hello. I hope you're well, and I hope you'll write back."

To which she responded: "You seem like pretty normal. Want to meet for dinner?"

To which I responded: "I *am* pretty normal. Except for the whole eating-human-flesh thing, but that was a *very* long time ago, and I *really* didn't like it, and my parole officer and I both agree that it's time to move on with my life."

I smiled, then deleted that message.

Instead, I responded: "Are you free this Friday night? If you don't mind coming into Manhattan, there's an Italian restaurant on 48th Street and Eighth Avenue called Ciro. We can meet there at 6:30."

To which she responded: "Sounds like a plan."

To which I responded: "I'll make the reservation."

So that was that.

Pamela from Secaucus was nothing if not prompt. Six twenty-nine was forty-five seconds old when she came bounding up Eighth Avenue. She recognized me and began to wave at a distance of half a block and shouted past roughly a dozen pedestrians, "Hey, you look just like your photos!"

Roughly a dozen pedestrians turned to ascertain the truth of her observation. I only shrugged at them.

"Is that good or bad?" I said as she got closer.

She didn't answer but rushed up to me and gave me the kind of hug more often reserved for POWs released from years of captivity. Then she stepped back and spun around. "So what about me?"

"You look very pretty," I said.

"But do I look like my photo?"

This, I sensed, was a trick question. She didn't look very much like her photo. Her hair was dark brown rather than blond, her facial features blunter, and there was noticeably more heft to her frame. Still, in the diminishing sunlight, and at certain angles, it became clear that the woman standing in front of me was indeed occupying the same physical space as Pamela from Secaucus.

"Yeah, you do," I said.

"You're a liar!" she shouted, then began to snort with laughter . . . and then punched me, hard, in the chest. "But I love you for it!"

Pamela hooked her arm around mine, and the two of us headed into Ciro. I nodded at the host—I'd been there often enough that he knew me by sight—and we were seated, as Flip Wilson's Geraldine character used to say, in a booth in the back in the corner in the dark.

"You know what attracted me to you?" she said, as soon as we got the menus.

"My punctuation?"

That made her snort again. I hadn't appreciated how loud that snort was when I'd heard it outside. It had the approximate report of an M-80 firecracker. The sound caused at least a dozen diners' heads to spin in our direction, like a scene out of *Children of the Damned.*

She said, "I was attracted to you because you don't wear a baseball cap."

"It's one of my best features."

That elicited another snort. "You're a *riot*!"

"Except I *do* wear a baseball cap occasionally."

"Yeah, but you don't use it to hide the fact that you're bald. Not that you're bald. But let's face it, you don't have a lot of hair. But you're not trying to hide anything. That tells me you're comfortable with yourself. You're not pretending to be something you're not. Most of the guys you meet on dating sites are such *fakes*. It makes me sick. That's why I like trannies. They keep it real."

"Trannies?"

"You know, *trannies*. Transvestites."

The waiter arrived at that moment to take our orders, and I told him we needed another minute to look at the menu. As Pamela was scanning down the list of entrees, I was working on a safe comeback to her theory of transvestites keeping it real. It was like a low-hanging Rubik's Cube. There were too many innuendos and too many moving parts.

I stared at the menu until the writing began to blur.

The waiter returned after a (very long) minute and smiled expectantly at us.

"Do you mind if I order wine?" she said.

"Not at all," I replied, grateful for the change of subject.

She glanced up at the waiter. "What would you recommend?"

He said the Shiraz went well with the Risotto Alla Pescatora, the dinner special. She nodded at both suggestions. Then I ordered baked ziti and a Diet Coke, and he bowed at the waist and left us alone.

"Sorry," I said, "I've never been much of a drinker—"

"Yep," she said, "I *loves* me my trannies."

"I've always liked Diet Coke better than Coke classic . . . and don't get me started on New Coke—"

"Do you want to see pictures?"

"Of what?"

"Me and my trannies," she said.

"All right . . ."

She fished her cell phone out of her purse, called up a photo album (conveniently labeled "Me and My Trannies") and handed it across the table. The album contained four photos of Pamela from Secaucus, mugging for the camera, surrounded by a half dozen transvestites in silk corsets and torpedo bras outside a lingerie shop in the West Village. The snow in the background indicated the shots were taken in the dead of winter. The last one featured Pamela, on her knees, about to perform fellatio on one of her friends, holding the shaft of his penis, while the rest laughed and applauded.

"Wow," I said, handing back the phone.

"Are you shocked?"

"Who, me? Nah."

"I didn't suck him off, in case you're jealous. That was just a gag photo."

If there is a clever, or even satisfactory, rejoinder to that remark, I couldn't come up with it (and haven't been able to come up with it in the years since). I was rescued, however, by the reappearance of our waiter with the glass of Shiraz. He set it down in front of her, and she lifted it up to her nose and sniffed. Then she lifted the glass to eye level and rolled the wine round and round. She studied it intently as the waiter and I watched her.

Then she looked up at the waiter and snapped her fingers. "Take it away."

"Don't you want to taste it?"

"I don't drink swill!"

The same dozen diners as before turned in our direction.

"Very good," the waiter said. "May I bring you something else?"

"Just bring me the house wine," she said, "and in a clean glass!"

So my ziti will be served with waiter's spit, I thought.

"I'm sorry about that," Pamela said. "I'm a total wine snob."

The words registered, and I nodded at them. But a sudden, peculiar calm had come over me. My date with Pamela of Secaucus had become like a bad ride at an amusement park. It wasn't going to kill me. I just had to wait it out. It was an hour out of my life, and it would end, and I'd walk away intact. Of course I could never go back to Ciro. But there were other Italian restaurants on the West Side. *Que sera, sera.*

"No reason to apologize," I said, smiling. "You know what you like."

"I do!"

"It shows."

"I've taken classes," she said. "The grapes speak to me. I *get* them."

"It's a conversation."

"*Exactamundo*."

The waiter returned with another glass, this one empty, and a bottle of wine in the crook of his elbow. He set the glass down on the table and poured in a sip of wine for her to taste. Again, she rolled the glass around and lifted it to eye level. She drank the sip and swished it around in her mouth. I thought, for a split second, she was going to drool it back into the glass. But she swallowed it. The slightest hint of a smile came over her face. Then she snapped her fingers twice and pointed to the glass. The waiter filled up the glass and walked away.

"You can't let them walk all over you," she explained.

"Of course not."

"The only reason they can get away with stuff is because people are intimidated."

"But not us," I said.

"You're being sarcastic, aren't you?"

"Who, me?"

The food arrived, so she didn't have to respond. The waiter lingered as she tasted her risotto. She took a small bite, shrugged in an "I've had worse" kind of way, and the dozen diners in our immediate vicinity collectively exhaled. I started in on my spit-laced ziti, and then, for a long time, neither of us spoke.

She broke the silence after several minutes. "Can I put something on the table?"

"What do you mean?" I said.

She set down her silverware and looked me in the eye. "I don't think this is going anywhere."

"*This?*"

"The two of us."

"Oh."

"I mean, I'll fuck you if you want. But, long term, I don't see us together."

"I agree," I said.

She smiled. "Then we probably shouldn't fuck."

"Yeah, I'm thinking that would be a mistake."

"You're a nice guy," she said. "I mean it."

"That's my curse."

"Are you sure you don't want a blowjob?"

"You're testing me, aren't you?"

"Yeah, and you passed," she said.

"What's my reward?"

"Do you want a blowjob?"

That cracked me up, genuinely, and for the rest of the meal we bantered back and forth. Knowing that we'd never see one another again, and knowing that we both knew it made for a downright pleasant second half of the date. It occurred to me as I was paying the check that I *liked* Pamela from Secaucus—that, if I weren't such a damned nice guy, I'd be proud to get a blowjob from her.

We parted, with a firm handshake, on the corner of West 48th Street. Watching her saunter off in the direction of the Port Authority Bus Terminal, I came to a realization about online dating—the truth of which would be underscored again and again as I shotgunned through profiles on eHarmony and other websites over a period of several years: Many of us, myself no doubt included, make our best impressions when we're not actually there.

THE BALLET WORKOUT

I am lying on my back. Sweat is trickling from my temples through the curls of hair above my ears, around to the back of my neck, and then dripping onto the vinyl mat. My left leg is bent at the knee; my right leg is wrenched across my left leg to form the number 4. My left hand is stretching through the hole of the 4 and pulling my right leg forward, grasping in vain for my right hand behind my right thigh.

Literally, I am tying myself in a knot.

It's not what I had in mind when I signed up for The Ballet Workout. The idea originated last fall with Sal, the player-manager of one of my softball teams, toward the end of another injury-riddled season. I pulled my hamstring for the ninth time in six years, then pulled a groin muscle compensating for the hamstring, then pulled a muscle below my rib cage sneezing. Maybe, Sal said, I ought to work on flexibility. He suggested yoga. But I've always held a dim view of yoga, of the in-your-face serenity of its practitioners, as though the ability to twist your leg behind your head translated into enlightenment.

The Ballet Workout seemed more likely. For one thing, it wasn't an *actual* ballet class, so I wouldn't have to wear tights or dance slippers. For another, I'd once briefly dated a woman who taught me the five basic foot positions, so I figured I already had a leg up. Besides, I'd been told several times that I looked graceful playing center field . . . so I thought maybe I'd turn out to be a natural, that I'd end up doing spinny Baryshnikov things from one end of the studio to the other.

That image lasted five minutes into the first session. It lasted five minutes only because Anna, the instructor, was four minutes late. The class consisted of nine women and me, and as we waited for her to arrive, I watched myself in the mirror. I *looked* like a dancer. I was wearing a sleeveless gray tee shirt, black bicycle shorts and a light blue bandanna tied across my forehead. Rolling my head from side to side, loosening up, I noticed the stark overhead light shadowing my high Bolshoi cheekbones.

Finally, Anna entered the room. She was a petite woman with dark brown hair, very pretty, in her late twenties. She walked up to me at once and glanced down at my feet.

"You might want to lose those."

She meant my Chuck Taylor high-tops.

While I unlaced the sneakers, Anna stepped to the front of the class and called out, "Warm-ups."

The rest of the class collected vinyl mats from the corner and then slid down onto them, and I followed their lead—thankful that neither of my socks had a hole in the toe. As we shifted from one side to another, rotating our legs at odd angles to loosen our hip joints, I still felt vaguely adequate. The first real trouble came when we rolled onto our stomachs. Anna told us to extend our right leg and left arm; this I managed by pressing my forehead into the mat for a kind of tripod balance. A moment later, I heard Anna's voice above me. "Head back! Head back! That's right. Now chin up!"

The instant I pulled my chin up, I keeled to the left, banging my high left Bolshoi cheekbone onto the edge of the mat and wood floor. I glanced up at Anna, forcing a smile, a signal that only my dignity was hurt. We reversed arms and legs, then back again, back and forth. The rest of the class was flexing and arching, a flock of swans; I was a buckshot goose stiffening with rigor mortis.

Next, we rolled onto our backs. "Hands beneath your rear ends," Anna shouted, assuming the position herself, "small of your back pressed into the mat, legs straight up in the air, feet turned out . . . now your legs come apart."

All right, I had my hands beneath my rear end.

"Legs up in the air," she called to me. "*Up* in the air. *Way* up. Straight knees! Straight knees! That's right. Now your legs come apart. Just let them fall apart."

Reluctantly, my legs drifted apart: *Got it*, I thought.

Then I peered at Anna in front of the room. Her legs were extended to a clock position of three forty-five. I glanced up at mine: ten minutes to two.

"Now legs together!"

I brought mine together.

"Now back apart . . . see if you can go further."

I was still at ten to two: Anna was now at four forty.

As we continued our floor work, straightening and rounding, coiling and relaxing, I came to realize that she was boneless, a cross between a woodland sprite and Gumby. She was doing things with her body that I couldn't have done if I'd been able to step out of my skeleton and twist from the outside. Still, Anna managed an occasional smile in my direction. I was pleased, too, that none of the other students seemed to notice how awkward I felt. They were too focused on keeping up with Anna's instructions.

After several more minutes on the mats, Anna told us to stand up and catch our breaths. When I glimpsed myself in the mirror, what a change I saw! I had sweated through the back and sides of my gray tee shirt, and my hair was soaked into ringlets that lined the rim of the bandanna.

The woman next to me whispered, "Good workout."

"Is it over?"

She laughed softly.

"Feet in first position!" Anna called.

That, I knew I how to do: knees straight, heels together, toes turned out to 180 degrees. Anna nodded in approval as I teetered for an instant, then steadied myself.

"Now, *demi-plié* . . ."

As the words left her mouth, Anna sank in a perfect line toward the floor, her feet still opposed, her heels still together, her thighs and calves diamonding out, her arms billowing at her sides; a second later, she rose again to her full height, her knees straightening, her arms rolling upward at the same pace as her torso. The movement was breathtaking in its simplicity and grace. I watched her do another, then, on her third call, attempted my first *demi-plié*.

"Good!" she said.

I nodded to her: *No problem.*

"Now, with me, on the beat . . . *plié* . . . *plié* . . . *plié* . . ."

The word itself became the count, the forceful *plee* the dip, the breathless *yeh* the rise. For a half dozen *pliés*, I was keeping up, adapting to the cadences of her voice. The two of us were partners, bodies in motion together. But then, accidentally, I glimpsed myself in the mirror. The truth hit hard. I was not Anna's partner. I was a dancing bear. No, I was one of those Ray Harryhausen clay dinosaurs that lurch between frames of film. The hunch in my shoulders as I curled my arms was australopithecine.

"Right leg brushes forward and back! Foot pointed! Now . . . brush . . . brush . . . brush . . ."

I watched my right foot swinging forward and back. I was determined not to look in the mirror again. My balance was shaky. I wobbled on my left leg twice, but I continued to brush. For the remainder of the class, I sank back into myself, focused on Anna's directions, mimicked her movements half-heartedly. What I wanted, throughout, was to be back in center field, circling underneath a fly ball, doing something I was good at—and I wanted Anna sitting in the bleachers. Watching me. Waving at me. Nodding her head.

When the class ended, I hurried out. *Never again*, I thought. That resolution intensified the following morning: I ached in places I'd never ached before, felt spasms where I didn't know I had muscles. Still, as the week wore on, I began to waver. The aches faded, the spasms petered out. I was left with the recognition that ballet was the first physical activity I'd ever been bad at. Sure, I'd been mediocre at lots of things, but never *bad*. I began to feel for those kids in the playground—you know, the last picks of the pickup games, the Rodneys and Sheldons and Iras, who seemed predestined to watch grounders dribble through their legs or pop-ups ricochet off their chests. *They* always came back. Week after week, praying perhaps that their bodies would start to follow their wills, that their mental images would come to match reality, that the recipe for athletic coordination would at last dawn on them.

Of course, it never did.

Nevertheless, that is my hope now as I return week after week to The Ballet Workout . . . that someday, somehow, suddenly, I will glance past Anna and into the mirror and see something that resembles a dancer.

MOVIES

I was never an avid moviegoer, not even when I was a teenager, when it was the thing to do on a Saturday night. Nowadays, in an average year, I'll see maybe two or three films in the theater. When I do venture out, there are three conditions upon which I insist:

First, *I will not see a movie on the night it opens.* I don't like crowds, and I especially don't like crowds comprised of the kind of people who feel the need to see a movie before anyone else does. Such crowds tend to be younger and rowdier than should be gathered under a single roof, or at least gathered under a single roof without a nun with a ruler to keep order. They tend to yell advice at the characters on the screen, then to shush one another for yelling advice at the characters on the screen, and then to challenge one another to fist fights for shushing one another.

Second, *I will not sit anywhere except on the aisle.* In a controlled environment—say, on the sofa in my living room—I can easily sit through a two-hour movie without having to get up and use the bathroom. However, the bladder has a mind of its own; if it senses that a bathroom break cannot be had, or can be had only by climbing over the scrunched-in knees of a half dozen cranky strangers, it will fill up again and again, in defiance of mammalian probabilities, as if to reprimand its owner for putting it in such a precarious situation.

Third, *I will not see a Leonardo DiCaprio movie.* Leo and I have a bad history, going back to 1996 when he starred in *William Shakespeare's Romeo + Juliet*. I was running on a treadmill in the gym, listening to FM radio through a headset plugged into the treadmill's entertainment unit, when I heard an ad for the film. It sounded like the kind of thing I'd want to see, like the kind of thing I might even want to show to my freshman English class in lieu of Franco Zeffirelli's stuffy '68 version of the play. The new version, apart from Leo, also starred Clare Danes—whose name I recognized from MTV's *My So-Called Life*. I could well imagine her as an angst-plagued Juliet. On the whole, I was feeling pretty enthusiastic about *R + J* right up until the ad ended, and I was urged to buy the soundtrack, which featured music from a band called the Butthole Surfers. I remember thinking, "What the hell?" . . . and then stumbling, ever so slightly, on the treadmill. The headphones jerked out of my ears, and I made a grab for them, which caused me to trip over my feet, fall onto my side, and shoot off the back of the treadmill, knocking over two young women in spandex outfits who'd been chatting behind me. As one witness said, it looked like I was picking up a six-ten spare.

Which leads me to the occasion I violated all three of my moviegoing rules—and vowed never to do so again. The year was 1997. I was dating Carmen, who, at certain angles, and in a certain light, resembled the actress Andie MacDowell (slightly relevant) and who was a diehard romantic (very relevant). Carmen got it into her head, weeks in advance, that she was going to see the movie *Titanic* the night it opened. Not that she *wanted* to see it. She was *going* to see it, with or without me.

Now I wasn't exactly wise in the ways of *amore*, but even I knew that you didn't let your new girlfriend, who kind of looked like Andie MacDowell, go alone to the decade's most romantic movie. Thus, on Friday morning, December 19, 1997, Carmen stood in line outside her local theater and bought two tickets as soon as the box office opened. The fact that there had been a line just to *buy* tickets *in the morning* was an ominous sign. So the two of us arrived at the theater that evening two hours in advance of the eight o'clock show and stood at the head of a line that eventually turned the corner and took up most of two New York City blocks. As the doors opened, Carmen rushed inside to claim our seats and dispatched me for a farm silo of popcorn, along with two barrels of Diet Coke.

For half a minute after I entered the theater itself I could not find her. Then at last I caught sight of a distant hand wave. She was dead center, front to back, and dead center, side to side. It was the side-to-side position that caused me to cringe. There were a dozen seats on either side of the two she'd staked out.

They were filling fast.

I negotiated the obstacle course between us without spilling a kernel of popcorn or a drop of soda—though I likely wouldn't have made it had not half the row stood up to let me pass. No one said a word, because the movie hadn't begun yet, but there were several glares. I handed Carmen the food and drink, then looked left and right; I knew at once there was no chance, none whatsoever, that I would be getting up from that seat until the movie was over.

That was the first inkling that I needed to pee.

I settled in for fifteen minutes of previews and hunkered down for the feature presentation. Toward the end of the opening credits, the fact that I had to use the facilities had begun to recede in my consciousness. There was no urgency, not yet, and I was soon caught up in the story, rooting hard for Jack (Leo) to make it onto the ship, sighing at the initial appearance of Rose (Kate Winslet), hissing at the entrance of Rose's boorish fiancé, Cal (Billy Zane). The first full-screen shot of the *Titanic* itself wowed me in a "that's entertainment" kind of way.

It was an hour into the movie, right around the time Jack begins to sketch Rose in the nude, that the need to pee pressed itself to the forefront of my mind. Again, I glanced to the left and to the right.

No way out.

All right, I thought, *here I am*. I shouldn't have gotten myself in this predicament, but I did, and there's nothing to do now except tough it out. Human beings have endured worse punishments than an hour or so of internal discomfort. Think of Robert De Niro and Christopher Walken in *The Deer Hunter*. Think of Sylvester Stallone in *Rocky IV*—

or the audiences who had to sit through *Rocky IV*. Think of Shemp stumbling into a tool shed. Compared with them, I had it pretty damn easy. Plus, I had an epic saga unfolding in front of me. That gigantic special-effected ocean liner was about to hit a digital iceberg and sink! I wasn't going to let a couple of hundred milliliters of distraction ruin the spectacle.

That was what I told myself.

Titanic runs three hours and fourteen minutes. The entire second half of the movie consists of running water—water crashing through the ship's hull and into the engine room, water filling the lower levels of the ship, corridor by corridor, water rushing up stairs and into staterooms. There's Jack, handcuffed to a steam pipe, as the water rises from his ankles to his waist to his chest; there's Rose, wading into the water to find Jack, her gown clinging to her heaving breasts, then making a swim for it until at last the drenched lovers are reunited. Then, of course, there is the ocean itself, the whirl and roil and crest of its waves.

Each scene, each shot, each frame, seemed to resonate within my bladder.

There are certain degrees of biological exigency that no leg-crossing can tame. The desire for relief and the will to uphold personal dignity go to war—the former in breakout mode, the latter in containment. It is a kind of homeostatic Battle of the Bulge, and I fought it, hammer and tongs, for two solid hours. By the end, my left leg was at my right hip in Half Lotus position, and my right foot was tapping the floor at a speed that approached a Buddy Rich drum solo. My heart was throbbing in my chest, and sweat was beading on my forehead.

If there had been a single laugh in the last half hour of the movie, I'd have been a goner.

But there wasn't . . . and when, at last, the aged Rose tossed that blue heart-shaped pendant over the side of the salvage ship, and when, at last, she and Jack were reunited in death, both youthful, both beautiful, gazing into one another's eyes on the polished marble stairwell of the revived *Titanic*, and when, at last, the credits began to roll, and the lights went on, and the theater filled with the voice of Celine Dion, I jumped up . . . only to be pulled back down by Carmen, who, like the rest of the audience, remained in their seats, applauding the name of producer/director/writer James Cameron, and then, one by one, the names of each of the principal actors. Only as the identities of the key grip and makeup artists were revealed did the crowd begin to exit the theater. By then I had slipped into a state of calm, almost euphoria, akin, I suspect, to what climbers feel on Everest when their bivouac has failed and when the chill of the mountain snow becomes one with their bones.

Then, at once, there was a path to the aisle . . . and then another path to the exit. I left Carmen blubbering in her seat and scrambled out. Sighting the men's room, I sprinted and shoved my way past men twice my size, their eyes moist with emotion, and thus mercifully oblivious to my cutting in front of them. Moments later, I was standing in front of the urinal.

Relief was at hand.

Then, for several seconds, nothing. The more colloquial term for such a pause is "stage fright," but this had more the feel of a lone Japanese soldier, decades after World War II has ended, holed up in his bunker on a remote South Pacific island, still wary of letting go, still believing, because he cannot quite believe otherwise, that the war rages on, that the fate of the Empire rests with him

But then, at long last, relief.

Carmen awaited me in the theater lobby, at the edge of the corridor that led to the restrooms. Her eyes were puffy and red, and she had a wad of balled-up tissues in her left hand. She had a tragic look on her face. It was a look I'd seen before.

I walked her home, and she kissed me on the cheek when we came to her door. Several days later, in a letter, she told me that she no longer wanted to continue our romance, that she had come to realize, watching the movie, that I didn't complete her, that I wasn't her soul mate, her one true love—the one she wanted by her side when the credits began to roll.

That metaphor has stuck with me through the years. For it caused me to realize that, despite the many ways in which we divide ourselves—by ethnicity, by creed, by gender and age and geography—when the final credits begin to roll, there really are only two tribes of human beings. Center People and Aisle People. Compared with these, other divisions are trivial. Carmen was center stock. I was aisle to the core. Therefore: My heart *would* go on without her.

So, too, would my bladder.

LETTUCE PREY

It was just after two in the morning on a Friday night, and I was six blocks from my Midtown apartment. I was carrying a pound and a half of sliced turkey in a Ziploc bag in my knapsack, the reward for staying to help friends clean up after their Christmas party. The fact that I was packing meat reminded me, as I passed a twenty-four-hour deli, that I needed groceries. So I angled into the store, picked up a half dozen items and turned for the cash register. But then I thought again about the pound and a half of turkey. Since I was going to be eating sandwiches for the next several days, I grabbed a head of iceberg lettuce and dropped it into my basket.

Waiting for a homeless man to count out a fistful of coins for a wine cooler, I did a quick estimate of what I was about to pay. Even though a couple of the items weren't marked, I guessed the total at ten dollars. When my turn came, I didn't watch as the cashier, a dark-skinned guy with a wispy goatee, rang up each item; only when he announced the sailed-the-ocean-blue total of fourteen dollars and ninety-two cents did I glance up.

"That can't be right," I said, smiling.

He rolled his eyes. Then he began to point at each item and state the price; he did this with much haste, but as he called out the numbers, I was doing the addition a second time in my head. Finally, he'd counted everything except the head of lettuce. The total I'd come up with, not including the lettuce, was a few cents shy of ten dollars.

He picked up the head of lettuce, then hesitated.

"How much is it?" I asked.

He smiled and said, "Four ninety-nine."

"Four ninety-nine? Isn't that a bit steep?"

"You want it or not?"

I began to waver. Four ninety-nine *seemed* like a lot to pay for a head of lettuce, but in truth I hadn't bought one since roughly the second Reagan administration, so I wasn't sure. For all I knew, there might've been a dire lettuce harvest, or perhaps a long and bitter strike by migrant workers, and prices had skyrocketed as a consequence. In any event, there were now three people in line behind me—I didn't want them to think that I was the sort of person who wouldn't pay the going rate for a head of lettuce.

So I reached into my wallet and plunked down fourteen dollars and ninety-two cents.

The cashier smiled again and said, "Have a nice night."

As I walked the six blocks home, the four ninety-nine head of lettuce began to prey on my mind. I was convinced I'd been deeply and deliberately gouged, but I hadn't asked for a receipt, so it was mine, for better or worse. I stopped and took it out of the bag. It was in fact a fine-looking head of lettuce—hefty but not leaden, rounded to a skullish symmetry, absent the inky brown gunk at the stem. Underneath its cellophane, it glistened in the streetlight. It occurred to me, as I admired it, that I now had an *investment*. So I made a quick detour. There was a twenty-four-hour Duane Reade three blocks away. There, I picked out a deep round faux Tupperware container for my lettuce. The cashier, a stocky black woman with cornrowed hair, regarded the purchase with perfect indifference . . . not a hint of curiosity as to the airtight emergency that had brought me to her register at two thirty in the morning. Too bad since, had she asked, I'd concocted an elaborate backstory in which I was delivering a heart for transplantation.

The faux Tupperware container set me back six dollars and ninety-nine cents, so I was into the head of lettuce for twelve bucks at this point. Rather than just rolling it into the crisper at the bottom of the refrigerator and falling into bed, I unwrapped it as soon as I got home. This I did with great care. I remembered that you were supposed to peel off the outer layer before you washed it, but this was no ordinary head of lettuce; I could not bring myself to waste any of it. I did peel off the outer layer and rinsed the head itself, but once I had it secured inside the faux-Tupperware container and stored in the crisper, I rinsed off the outer layer and ate it, with a sprinkling of salt, as a late-night snack.

It was delicious.

When I woke up Saturday morning, I stumbled into the kitchen and reached for my usual breakfast: an unfrosted strawberry Pop-Tart. But then I thought about the lettuce. It was now one night old. I was pretty sure I'd never owned a head of lettuce that I had finished; always, it had gone bad before I got down to the core. So I pulled the faux-Tupperware container out of the refrigerator, took out the lettuce, and peeled off another layer. Then I set the layer between two slices of white bread. It was the first lettuce sandwich I'd ever eaten. Just lettuce and bread.

It was delicious.

For lunch, I had a turkey and lettuce sandwich, then added Swiss cheese and mustard to the mix for dinner. Afterward, I watched a college football game with the faux-Tupperware container in my lap, snacking on shards of lettuce as though they were potato chips. That night, before I turned in, I took a last look at the head of lettuce. About a third of it was gone. I felt as though I was making good progress.

Sunday morning, however, I was discouraged to find that the lettuce had begun to wilt. I had to discard the new outer layer, which had the texture and consistency of rose petals. I ate another lettuce sandwich for breakfast—which, tinged with a sudden urgency, seemed even sweeter than the one from the morning before. I could not recall a tastier breakfast; I felt invigorated by it, cleansed body and soul. For lunch, I had a plain lettuce salad with Italian dressing and another turkey and lettuce sandwich. Then, for dinner, I had two more turkey-and-lettuce sandwiches . . . which exhausted the sliced turkey I'd taken home from the Christmas party.

Less than a third of the lettuce remained when I turned in on Sunday night. I was going to do this thing; I was going to finish the head of lettuce. What's more, I *liked* the lettuce. It was low in calories and cholesterol, rich in potassium, a veritable tonic for many of the arterial diseases that befall Semites later in life. As I lay in bed, I began to think of the money I'd save if I made myself two salads per day instead of the usual slice of pizza for lunch and Chinese takeout for dinner . . .

Then, at once, I sat up in bed. Was *that* what the last three days were all about? Money? Had I worked up a sudden passion for an otherwise indifferent leafy vegetable, a leafy vegetable I habitually left over whenever it turned up next to a burger and fries, or on a plate of cheese enchiladas, only because in the back of my mind I knew I'd grossly overpaid for it? I felt like Shylock. The head of lettuce had become the better part of my affections.

In a spasm of self-hatred, I threw back the covers, rushed out of the bedroom and into the kitchen. I yanked open the refrigerator and grabbed the faux-Tupperware container with the last third of the lettuce, tore off the lid, and dumped the contents into the garbage can. The gesture still did not suffice. With my heart racing, I snatched the garbage bag from the plastic can and carried it down the hall to the compactor room. Only as I shoved the garbage bag down the chute did I feel altogether rid of the head of lettuce.

Then, at last, I went back to bed.

Unfortunately, I woke up Monday morning craving lettuce. I tried to talk myself out of it, toasted a Pop-Tart out of habit. But after a couple of bites, I couldn't finish it. There was no denying the fact that I wanted a lettuce sandwich. I got dressed and headed downstairs to the local Food Emporium. There, I picked out a fine head of lettuce for one dollar and forty-nine cents—which confirmed, once and for all, that I'd been overcharged at the twenty-four-hour deli. I peeled off the outer layer as soon as I got home and washed the rest, then ripped off a hunk and set it between two slices of white bread.

It had no taste. None whatsoever.

I stared down at the half-eaten sandwich in disbelief. It did not seem possible that such a difference could exist between two members of the iceberg family. Perhaps I'd chosen a poor specimen? So I went back out and bought another. It was on special sale for one dollar and twenty-nine cents at Gristedes nine blocks to the west. I brought it home, washed it, broke off a piece, and ate it plain.

Again, nothing.

Out of desperation, I went back out a third time . . . back to the twenty-four-hour deli at which I'd been gouged for the first head of lettuce. There was a different cashier now, a young Asian guy in a Yankees tee shirt and jeans, and he rang up the new lettuce for one dollar and ninety-nine cents.

"You know," I said, "I paid four ninety-nine for a head of lettuce here Friday night."

He smiled at me and said, "That's not possible."

"I did."

"You got a receipt?"

I shook my head.

He smiled at me and shrugged.

The new lettuce, when I got it home, had the same non-taste as the two I'd bought that morning. For several minutes, I weighed the likelihood that the first head of lettuce had been an aberration, a sui generis expression of Frostian elements—sun and soil, leaf and dew—that had fallen into my lap. But I was compelled, in the end, to accept that the difference wasn't in the lettuce; it was in me. Knowing that I'd overpaid for that first head of lettuce made it taste better.

No two ways about it: I was a Semitic stereotype.

Now I stared at the heads of wasted lettuce, three anatomies of melancholy, lined up along the kitchen counter, and I thought about the remnants of that first head of lettuce, smothered in soot at the bottom of the compactor chute. To what end?

Many years ago, a friend of mine named Danny suggested that another friend, who'd recently gotten engaged, wasn't happy. "He only thinks he's happy because she's his first girlfriend," Danny said. "Just wait a year and see what happens." The fact that the marriage lasted less than a year seemed at the time to vindicate Danny's point. But now I'm not so sure. Is there a difference between *thinking* you're happy and *being* happy? Temporary happiness, after all, is still happiness.

Likewise, is there a difference between *thinking* you like lettuce and *liking* lettuce? Pleasure in the mind is pleasure, plain and simple. Tom Sawyer tricks his buddies into believing that he enjoys whitewashing a fence; they wind up bribing him to take turns doing his job for him. But if Tom has convinced them that whitewashing the fence is enjoyable, and if indeed they're enjoying themselves whitewashing the fence, then Ben Rogers and Billy Fisher and Johnny Miller have no gripe against Tom. They've gotten fair value.

So what's the moral of my lettuce tale? Maybe just that analysis is occasionally the enemy of pleasure—as anyone who's ever studied literature in graduate school will confirm. Now and then the wiser course is to accept the thing at face value. To take it for what it is.

Especially if it's rich in potassium.

MY LAST VISIT TO DOCTOR B

I'd been sick off and on for over a month with flu-like symptoms when my ex-girlfriend Linda recommended, in her gentle way, that perhaps I ought to see a physician. "You're *going* to the doctor," she told me, as she delivered a carton of orange juice to my apartment for the third time in a week.

Her words irked me . . . or at least her words *would* have irked me if an irk could have penetrated the steel-wool cobweb of mucous and fever gathered behind my face. Linda had consistently ordered me around during the two years that we lived together, but now that we'd parted, I saw no reason to acquiesce. So I narrowed the one eye I could open at her and said, "I'm *not* going to the doctor."

To which she replied, "Oh, you're *going* to the doctor."

So I made an appointment with Doctor B for the following afternoon.

Now I should mention, by way of background, that Doctor B was not a very good doctor. He was kindhearted and well-meaning, but disorganized to an unprofessional degree, forgetful to an unnerving degree, and deaf to a classifiable degree—and the respective degrees only worsened as he grew older. He was now in his mid-eighties. If you want to picture him, imagine the Phantom of the Opera, unmasked but not unpleasant, underneath a shock of jet-black Ronald Reagan hair. He had been my doctor for ten years. I kept going back to him because he had an office on the seventy-seventh floor of the Empire State Building, so sitting in his waiting room was an event, a mere nine floors shy of the eighty-sixth floor observatory. Occasionally, I'd bring a pair of binoculars and arrive a half hour before my checkup to take in the view.

That Thursday afternoon, however, I was in no condition to sightsee. My nose was running so profusely that I could not take the handkerchief from in front of my face long enough even to sign in. My throat was raw from coughing, and my left eye felt as if an interrogator had his thumb in it and was pressing, hard, to find out what I knew.

Ten minutes after arriving, I was led by Nurse Angela from the waiting area to Doctor B's office.

He did not realize at first that I'd sat down across the desk from him. He continued to shuffle through papers until he found my folder, and then he opened the folder and sifted through its contents, shaking his head from side to side. Then at last he looked up and called out, "Nurse, send in Mr. Goldb—" He startled at the sight of me, then continued, "Wait, never mind, he's here. . . . You look like crap."

"Yeah," I managed. "It's a recurring cold or maybe a flu."

"How long have you had it?"

"Off and on, maybe a month."

"You got colored mucous?"

"Yes."

"What colors?"

"Many colors."

"Sounds like a sinus infection," he said. "I'll give you an antibiotic. Should knock it right out of you."

I rubbed my nose with the soaked handkerchief. "Thank you."

"I notice you haven't been here in four years."

"I don't think it's been that long," I said.

"No, it says right here. I saw you in November 2005. That's the last time."

"I think—"

"We're going to have to do some blood work on you."

"Can't we put that off for another time—"

"No, wait," he said, shuffling the papers again. "I was wrong. You were here in 2006 . . . oh, and 2007 . . . and 2008. You were here twice in 2008."

"That's what I thought—"

"But you missed 2009."

"It must have skipped my mind."

"Just to be safe, we'll do the blood work on you."

I lowered my head in defeat. "Whatever you say."

"Did you fast?"

"What?"

"Did you fast before you got here?"

"No."

He made a note that I hadn't fasted.

Doctor B dismissed me, and I staggered down a long, narrow corridor lined with half-opened file cabinets, stacks of corrugated boxes, a teetering coat rack, a macaroni-and-cheese-stained microwave oven, and a dilapidated coffee maker and, at last, into another room for the blood work. As Nurse Angela was poking at my left arm, searching for a likely vein, Doctor B reappeared waving a slip of paper. "I'm going to put you on amoxicillin for six days. Whatever you have, that should knock it right out of you. I'll see you a week from today to go over the results of the blood work."

That was my next-to-last visit to Doctor B.

My last visit to Doctor B came when I went back for the test results. As predicted, the amoxicillin had knocked the sinus infection out of me, and I was tempted to blow off the follow-up appointment. If there were something wrong in the blood work, I figured Doctor B would've called and told me. But Linda pointed out that he might not; given how I'd described his office, he might've lost the results under a pile of papers. She had a good point, or a reasonable point, or at least a point, which meant I was going back to Doctor B regardless, so I nodded and told her I would. To which she added, "Oh, and you've never had a colonoscopy. Ask him about that too."

By the following Thursday, when I returned for the test results, I was feeling like a new man, so I showed up early for my five fifteen appointment and claimed a window seat in the waiting room. From the seventy-seventh floor of the Empire State Building, the northern half of Manhattan resembles a giant ship run aground against the southwest edge of the Bronx. There were water taxis angling from the Jersey shore across the Hudson toward the pier at Thirty-Ninth Street; to the east, traffic was crawling across the Queensborough Bridge. The spire of the Chrysler Building was glistening in the waning sunlight.

Nurse Angela interrupted my reveries and led me back to Doctor B's office. He was looking up this time as I entered. He smiled broadly at me and said, "Knocked it right out of you, didn't it?"

"Yes, it did," I said, taking a seat.

"Good old amoxicillin. Can't beat the stuff."

"I'm very grateful . . ."

But he was already flipping through the results of the blood work from the previous week. "Now let's see what's what. Your cholesterol is so-so, and I'm not crazy about the ratio of good to bad. You've got a history of that though, and it's not getting worse, so for the time being, we'll just monitor it. What else? Okay, here, it looks like your triglycerides are off the chart. But I wrote a note that says you didn't fast before the blood test. Did you fast?"

"No."

"Why not?"

"I was sick," I said. "I didn't know I was going to have a blood test."

"Yeah, yeah, that's right. So we'll monitor that too for the time being."

"All right."

He flipped to the next page. "Okay, your testosterone is slightly low . . ."

I leaned forward for an explanation, but none came. Doctor B continued to scan down the report.

After several seconds, I asked, "Is that a problem?"

He looked up from the report. "What?"

"Is that a problem?"

"Is what a problem?"

"You just said I had low testosterone."

"*Slightly* low," he said, then looked back at the report.

"Should I worry about it?"

He glanced up again, faintly smiling. "You married?"

"No," I said.

"Do you have trouble getting erections?"

"Not as far as I can tell."

"What?"

"It's not a problem."

"Whether it's a problem or not, you don't have to live with it." He reached into the top drawer of his desk and pulled out a thick prescription pad. "Here, just take this to the Duane Reade downstairs—"

I began waving my hands. "No, no."

He looked up from the pad with irritation. "Do you want the prescription or not?"

"It's not a problem," I repeated.

"Why would it be a problem? I've already got the pad out."

"No, I meant it's not an issue."

"What?"

"There's no issue," I said with more force.

"You don't ejaculate?"

"What?" I said.

"You get erections, but there's no issue?"

"No!"

"Then what's the problem?"

"I have no problem getting erections! I have no problem ejaculating!" The instant I finished yelling, I could hear the words echoing down the hall, past the nurses' station and into the crowded waiting room.

Doctor B smiled. "Well, that's all to the good."

He made a note in the margin of the report and then continued to read. He came to the end moments later. I thought he was about to dismiss me, and I began to wonder whether I could somehow slink past the nurses' station and mail in my fifteen-dollar copay.

"So you're doing all right?" he said.

"Yes."

"You're in a committed relationship?"

"What?" I said.

"Just because you don't hear about AIDS the way you used to doesn't mean it's going away. It's still out there. It's still a threat."

"I don't think I'm at much of a risk."

"Don't be cocky about it!" he said. "Even if you're in a committed relationship, you're still at risk."

I nodded my head to humor him. "I'll keep that in mind."

But then that faint smile came back. "So how long have you known?"

"Known what?"

"You know . . ."

"I'm not sure—"

"You're gay."

"What?"

"I mean, did you know it all along, or did you figure it out later in life?"

For a split second, I weighed my options. If I corrected him, I'd get drawn deeper into a conversation I desperately wanted to end. If I let it pass, he'd likely make another note on my report. "I guess I figured it out late in life."

"How late?" he said.

"Very late."

"But you're okay with it now, right?"

"Yes."

"Because it's a different world out there. We're not living in the fifties anymore."

"Yes, I know. It's a relief."

"So what's the guy's name?"

"What guy?"

"You said you were in a committed relationship," Doctor B said. "What's his name?"

There was no turning back now. I looked him square in the eyes and said, "Alex."

"Where'd you meet him?"

"We met in a bookstore. In the fiction section."

Doctor B nodded. "He makes you happy?"

"Yes, he does," I said.

"That's nice. That's good to hear."

As Doctor B continued to smile and nod, the fact that I would have to change doctors, that I wouldn't be able to remember the details I was inventing, dawned on me. It came as a relief, truthfully. Knowing that I'd never again have to wade through the crowds of tourists in front of the Empire State Building when I felt sick. Knowing that I'd never again have to wait in line in the lobby for a security pass. Sure, it would be a pain to find a new doctor; there would be pages and pages of forms to fill out. But the break was going to happen.

No regrets, I thought.

So I smiled back at Doctor B and said, "He completes me."

"Then you hold on to him."

"I'll do that," I said.

Doctor B stood up a moment later and thrust out his hand. He was still smiling as I clasped his hand and shook it. I don't know if he recognized something in my expression, or if he was only being polite, but his last words to me were, "You just be happy. That's what matters."

Not the worst medical advice I've gotten.

HERTZ A LOT

The misadventure began, as most misadventures do, with a lightbulb-bright idea . . .

I was in Orlando, Florida, for a book event. My novel *Twerp* had been chosen as the "summer read" (the book assigned over the summer) at the Lake Highland Prepratory School—in part, I suspect, because I was one of the few living authors willing to endure the heat and humidity of central Florida in late August for a book event.

The trip, up until the Sunday in question, had gone well: I'd worn my new sweat-wicking underwear and spent three days (my upper limit) visiting relatives in West Palm Beach. Then, late Sunday morning, I'd driven the three hundred miles to Orlando in a rented Nissan Altima. I was scheduled to meet with the Lake Highland students the next day, Monday, and fly back to New York City that same evening. Monday, in other words, was going to be a (literally) eventful day. Thus, my lightbulb-bright idea: If I returned the rental car to Hertz on Sunday, when I had oodles of free time, rather than on Monday, when I'd be in full chicken-with-head-cut-off mode, I could reduce stress. Of course, that meant I'd be without a car on Monday. But I could take a taxi from the hotel to the school, and then from the school to the airport, and not worry about navigating the highways and streets of a strange city. I actually said the words, "What could go wrong?" under my breath when the lightbulb switched on.

That should've tipped me off.

I dropped off my luggage at the Courtyard Marriott, got directions from the hotel concierge to the nearest Hertz lot and was back out on the backstreets of Orlando in ten minutes, looking for 139 South Orange Avenue. To my great relief, after only one wrong turn, I found myself cruising along South Orange Avenue, with the address numbers increasing inexorably toward 139. It was another "What could go wrong?" moment. I felt home-free.

Except then the addresses jumped from 125 South Orange Avenue to 155 South Orange Avenue. No number 139. No telltale yellow Hertz sign. No trace of a rental lot anywhere in the vicinity.

I circled the block again . . . again, nothing.

So I circled a third time . . . again, nothing.

I would have circled a fourth time, but I was shamed by the memory of Albert Einstein's definition of madness: "doing the same thing over and over again and expecting different results." I pulled to the curb and weighed the likelihood that Einstein had actually uttered those words, since roughly ninety-nine percent of quotes attributed to Einstein are bogus. (If you trust Facebook posts, Einstein also said, "Logic will only get you from A to B. Imagination will take you everywhere" and "Who let the dogs out? Who? Who? Who?") But whether Einstein defined madness as doing the same thing and expecting different results, or as arguing with Schrödinger over cat food recipes, circling the block repeatedly, and hoping number 139 materialized magically out of the ether, seemed like a pretty stupid thing to do.

The smart thing to do, I decided, was to get out of the car and search on foot for 139 South Orange Avenue. That way, I'd be able to ask passersby, maybe even the doorman of an adjacent building. (Doormen, in my experience, almost always know more than they let on.)

I stepped out of the car just as a police car rolled by. The cop in the passenger seat shouted, "You can't park there!"

I quickly shouted after him, "Do you know where 139 South . . ."

He was preemptively shrugging as the car rolled out of earshot.

So I couldn't leave the Altima where it was. I needed to find a metered parking space. I began to drive up and down side streets searching for one, but after five minutes I remembered that it was Sunday, so the parking meters were turned off; the chances of finding an empty space were vanishingly slim.

Still, I had a Plan B. On one of my earlier passes down South Orange Avenue, I'd noticed a couple of multi-level municipal garages, so I looped back around, located one of them between a movie theater and a business center, took a ticket at the entrance and drove up the steep ramp to the first level.

I circled hopefully, but there were no empty spaces on the first level.

I drove up another steep ramp to the second level.

I circled hopefully, but there were no empty spaces there either.

I drove up another steep ramp to the third level.

Lo and behold . . . the Hertz rental car lot!

To call the thing a "lot," however, is deceptive. It consisted of six yellow-lined parking spaces at the far end of the third level of the garage centered around a concrete pillar, also painted yellow, and a yellow kiosk—which was unmanned. I carefully steered the Altima into the one remaining Hertz space, pushed the dashboard button to shut off the engine, leaned back against the driver's seat, and exhaled.

I have to pause at this point to explain that the Altima was the first car I'd ever driven without an ignition key. To start the engine, you stepped on the brake and pushed the on-off button; to shut it down, you put the car in Park and pushed the button again. The only thing that resembled an ignition key was the "fob"—a word I'd always associated with old-fashioned pocket watches (and therefore also with oil barons and Monopoly characters). The fob consisted of a metal key ring on which hung a plastic tab with electronic signal buttons to open the doors and the trunk. When the Hertz attendant explained the system to me back in West Palm Beach, I was struck at once by its cleverness. It sounded foolproof. You *couldn't* lock the keys in the car because: 1) You couldn't lock the doors from the outside unless you had the fob with you; 2) If you forgot the fob inside the car, you couldn't lock the doors; and 3) *There were no keys.*

Which returns us to the Hertz lot on the third level of the municipal garage at 139 South Orange Avenue. As I said, I parked the Altima and pressed the button to turn off the engine. Then I stepped out of the car, locked the doors using the fob, and walked over to the after-hours drop off box . . . where you dropped off your fob. The drop-off box had a helpful checklist taped to it, the last item of which read, "Be sure to note the mileage of your vehicle."

I had not, as it happened, noted the mileage of my vehicle.

I walked back to the car, fobbed open the door, and scanned the dashboard for the odometer. Unfortunately, the odometer on the Altima isn't visible unless the engine is on. So I climbed back into the driver's seat, stepped on the brake, and pushed the on-off button. The green fluorescent digits of the odometer glowed on. I fished a pen out of my backpack and duly noted the mileage on the back of the rental agreement, then put away the pen, climbed out of the car, locked the doors, and headed back to the drop-off box. I read down the checklist one more time. Yes, I'd parked the vehicle in a designated Hertz space. Yes, I'd locked the doors. Yes, I'd noted the mileage. With a sense of satisfaction and finality, I dropped the fob into the box.

It was at the exact moment that the fob struck the bottom of the drop-off box that I realized I'd forgotten to turn off the engine of the car.

For several seconds, I just stared at the Altima. The engine was running, and I had no way to get back inside to press the on-off button. How long would it take to run out of gas? Well, the tank was slightly more than three-quarters full when I pulled into the space, so I did a few quick calculations in my head and figured the answer was roughly . . . a month.

I called the Hertz help line to explore my options; The operator told me I had two: 1) Put a note on the windshield for the Hertz attendant, walk away from the car (taking the chance that a thief might hear the engine running during the night, break the window and steal the car), and let the attendant deal with it Monday morning when he arrived at work and opened the drop-off box; 2) Call for emergency roadside assistance (and be charged eighty-six dollars), wait with the car until the AAA truck arrived, have the mechanic jimmy open the door, and then turn off the engine.

How long would it take, I inquired, for AAA to arrive?

Between a half hour and an hour, the operator replied.

"Fine," I said. "I'll pay the eighty-six dollars. Send the AAA truck to the Hertz lot at 139 South Orange Avenue."

"I'll put in the call right now," she said.

Then I hung up and waited.

And waited.

And waited.

Now I like an exhaust-filled municipal garage in Orlando in August as much as the next guy, but after the first couple of hours, my patience began to wear thin. So I called the Hertz help line again and asked what the delay was about. The operator—a different woman—put in a call to the AAA dispatcher, who put in a call to the truck. After five minutes of holding the line, I was informed that the AAA driver was lost . . . he couldn't find 139 South Orange Avenue.

"Tell him it's in the municipal garage," I said, "on the third level."

I was put on hold as the Hertz operator relayed the information to the AAA dispatcher, and the dispatcher relayed the information to the mechanic in the truck. Five more minutes passed, at which point, a male voice—I had no idea who it was—said, "Got it!"

Click and buzz.

So I waited.

And waited.

And waited.

I'd now been in the municipal parking garage for three hours, and my phone was running out of battery power. I called back the Hertz operator, and she called back the AAA dispatcher, and he called back the mechanic in the truck. After another five minutes on hold, the Hertz operator came back on the line to tell me that the mechanic was driving around and around on the third level of the municipal parking garage and couldn't find me.

"There's no one driving around and around on the third level of the municipal parking garage," I said. "I know that for sure because I've been standing here the entire time."

"Do you think he's lying?" she asked.

"All I can tell you is he's not here," I said. "Maybe he's on the second level and thinks it's the third level. Should I walk downstairs and look for him?"

"No, stay with the car."

"Why don't you give him my phone number?" I said. "Maybe if I speak to him directly—"

I was put on hold again. Five minutes later—which seemed to be their default unit of hold time—the Hertz operator came back on the line and said, "All right, he's got your number. You should hear from him in another min—"

Right then, I got a call-waiting signal.

"Got to go." I hung up on her and picked up the other call.

"Hello, Uncle Mark," my niece said. "I just want to know how your trip—"

"Got to go, Jessica—" I hung up on her.

The mechanic called a half minute later. "Hey, look, I'm on the third floor of the parking garage, and you're not here," he said. "I can't keep driving around in circles all afternoon."

"Well, I'm on the third floor too, and *you're* not *here*."

"Tell me what you're looking at," he said.

"Parked cars," I said. "Also, a yellow Hertz kiosk."

"I guarantee you there's no Hertz kiosk on the third floor of this parking garage."

That was when it dawned on me: "You're in the wrong municipal garage. There's another one on the next block."

"Jeez!"

"It's between the movie theater and the business center."

"Roger that," he said. "I'll be there in five minutes."

No one had ever said "roger that" to me before. It was a minor consolation as I continued to wait.

Ten minutes later, the AAA truck screeched around the corner of the third level of the municipal parking lot. The mechanic was waving out the window as he rolled up to the Hertz area.

"Wow, man!" he shouted. "Am I glad to see you!"

"Likewise," I called back.

He hopped out of the truck. "So you locked your keys in the car?"

"Not exactly."

I told him what had happened. I was struck by his professionalism as he listened. He didn't laugh once. He didn't even grin. He only nodded sympathetically. When I was done, he said, "Happens all the time."

"But not to me."

That cracked him up.

It turns out that the procedure for breaking into a locked car, without knocking out the driver's window, hasn't evolved much since the 1970s—when I used to practice, just for fun, on my mom's lime-green American Motors Rambler. You still have to find the rubbery connective tissue where the window meets the doorframe, wedge in something like a coat hanger and hook the latch that keeps the door locked. But the technology has advanced. The AAA guy whipped out a compression bladder and pump to create space between the window and doorframe, then reached for a pre-bent wire rod with a pre-formed hook to get at the latch. He had the car open in thirty seconds.

"Okay," he said, "you're good to go."

"Well, I don't exactly want to *go*."

"Then I guess you're good to stay."

I slid into the driver's seat and pressed the on-off button.

I climbed out of the car and pressed a twenty-dollar bill in the guy's hand.

"That's not necessary," he said.

"Consider it hush money."

He smiled and stashed the bill in his shirt pocket, then got back into his truck and drove off.

ME AND GLUTEN

Certain realms of human experiences do not lend themselves to polite exposition. The gastrointestinal, for example. Writing about food itself is fine—indeed, it's a cottage industry. Hunting and gathering. Preparing and arranging. Garnishing and serving. Great literature has been devoted to caloric intake: "*Beans, beans, they're good for your heart . . .*"

But our collective imagination seems to falter at the back of the throat. The muse, it would seem, doesn't swallow. Each of us knows there's a decidedly unpoetic process at the back end of ingestion akin to the workings of a Play-Doh Fun Factory, but we prefer not to dwell on it.

Until the moment we have to.

For me, that moment came as I rounded the turn from mid to late fifties (or *fiddies* as the kids, for reasons I can only guess at, say nowadays). AARP had just gathered up my vitals from God-knows-where and begun to send me personalized invitations to sign up. *Look, we've even included a trial membership card!*

These I took great pleasure in ripping in half and recycling before I walked away from the mailbox. *AARP? Are you kidding me? I still play touch football! Sure, I have to call time-out a couple of times during the game, sprint to the woods behind the west end zone and pee. But, dammit, I run post patterns! And I get open too—whether or not the guy guarding me has cathed that morning!*

Around the time I hit speed-limit age, however, things started happening inside my body. Bad things. Ugly things. Nauseous cramps came in slow, acidic waves, and strange, feral noises began to emanate from my innards. I would go into more detail, but the description would likely cause you to set down this book, shudder for several minutes, and take a long, hot shower.

After suffering with the condition for three months, and whining about it incessantly to friends and co-workers, I bowed to their collective wisdom and made an appointment with Doctor L, my primary care physician. She shuddered as I described my symptoms, then ducked out of the examining room. (Perhaps to take a long, hot shower.) When she returned, she asked if I'd ever had a colonoscopy. I confessed that I hadn't. So she referred me to an affiliated gastroenterologist, Doctor P.

I phoned Doctor P's office as soon as I got home and made an appointment for my first colonoscopy—in two weeks. His office emailed a prescription for something called GoLYTELY to my local pharmacy, which I picked up the following morning. Mission accomplished, I thought.

There were still two weeks before my appointment, however. During those two weeks, I discovered that pretty much anyone who's ever had a colonoscopy is anxious to talk about it. You want to strike up a conversation with a middle-aged man? Just utter the word "GoLYTELY"—which, it turns out, is the brand name of the preparatory fluid that clears out your bowels prior to the procedure. I must have heard a half dozen epic tales of the mystical power and medieval puissance of GoLYTELY.

"You ever use a laxative?" my friend Charles asked.

"Well, yes—"

"Forget about it. This is absolutely nothing like that."

"C'mon, it has to be a *little* like that."

"Yeah, and a firecracker is a *little* like an atom bomb because they both go pop."

The consensus seemed to be that the twenty-four hours before the colonoscopy—the daylong fast and the GoLYTELY-enabled "prep"—were awful, but that the procedure itself was unremarkable, and the lingering effects of the anesthetic were arguably worth the entire ordeal. I have to admit, I was intrigued.

GoLYTELY comes in powdered form at the base of a one-gallon canister, which looks like the kind of thing you'd tote back and forth to a service station if your car ran out of gas. You fill the canister to the brim with tap water, then shake it vigorously. (This can be dizzying after a daylong fast.) Flavor packets are also provided, which come in sealed plastic Kool-Aid-type pouches that are emptied into to the canister after the tap water. The flavor options are cherry, lemon-lime, or pineapple. I picked pineapple—and for that reason, I'll never be able to vacation in Hawaii. Once the flavoring has been added, the mixture is shaken vigorously again. (I was seeing tweeting birds at this point.) Then comes the not-as-easy-as-it-sounds stage of downing one full glass of the stuff every fifteen minutes until it's gone.

After each glass, I sat down at my desk and waited for The Event.

I waited . . . and waited . . . and waited . . .

Nothing happened.

After I downed the last glass, I called Charles and told him of my predicament.

"Really?" he said. "You drank the whole thing, and still *nada*?"

"I feel like I'm marinating in pineapple juice. But otherwise, yeah, nothing."

"Wow, that's impressive."

"It's not impressive! What if it doesn't . . . work?"

Between the words *doesn't* and *work*, the GoLYTELY kicked in. *Kicked in*, however, should be understood in the barnyard sense. Imagine a spooked mule making a loud "hee-haw" sound, lurching forward and then lashing out with its hind legs, striking you in the lower abdomen. What followed was a blur of evacuation. Maybe a half dozen times during the first hour, I rose from the toilet thinking, "All right, that's *got to be* it" . . . only to rush back a half minute later thinking, "Nope, that's not it." My mother used to tease me about the fact that I'd swallowed a loose button when I was a baby; I was certain, during the second hour, I heard it clink against the inside of the bowl. After three hours, I was no longer even stepping out of the bathroom. Between rounds, I'd just slide down onto the cool tile floor, where I'd rest on my side for the minute or so until the next summoning. The only intellectual takeaway, for me, from the hours I spent prepositioned in the vicinity of the bowl is that *ass* is a euphemism. When you get down to brass tacks, what you're working with is an *anus*.

But then, at once, and without warning, the ordeal was over. I remember the sensation of my lower lip against the cool tile floor, and then, the next moment, the woozy recognition that I could peel my lower lip off the cool tile floor and stand up. That, I did. I held on to the sink and took deep breaths. After another minute, I glanced in the mirror. With a three-day makeover, I could've passed for a corpse.

I pulled back the shower curtain and turned on the water. After I'd adjusted it to lukewarm, I stepped in. But I got wobbly as I was soaping myself, so I just sat down in the tub and let the spray wash over me. I reached forward and closed the drain until the water filled the tub.

I wallowed there until I fell asleep.

I don't remember climbing out of the tub and getting into bed. But that was where I woke up the following morning. I felt shockingly good, as if I'd been massaged from the inside out. I also felt light. I stepped onto the scale in the bathroom and saw a number I hadn't seen since my early twenties. I wasn't even hungry—though it had been a good thirty-six hours since my last full meal.

Linda had offered to take the cab ride with me to the gastroenterologist for the colonoscopy, but I was feeling so good that I phoned and told her to grab a few more hours of sleep. She'd still have to meet me after the procedure, because doctors don't release colonoscopy patients on their own recognizance—not because they can't stand up and walk out of the office but because they're liable to get sidetracked on their way home by the sound of distant Jefferson Airplane music. (Yeah, I was looking forward to those drugs.) So I left my house alone, flagged down a taxi, and wound up in Doctor P's office fifteen minutes early.

After a barrage of paperwork, I was led by a big-haired nurse to a treatment room, ordered to take off my clothes, and handed a hospital gown. She said, "The opening should be in the back."

"Should I tie it?"

She smiled. "If you want."

I stripped off my clothes, tied the gown in the back, and hopped on the examining table. I was then left alone for roughly five minutes, during which time I thought about my mortality and how much I loved barbecue potato chips, and I resolved, if I survived the procedure, to be a kinder person, and to eat more barbecue potato chips. Doctor P and a distressingly pretty young nurse then entered the room, and she asked me to untie my gown and roll onto my side. This I did. She stood near my head and made eye contact as Doctor P positioned himself at the business end of the table. I heard him say, "Are you comfortable, Mr. Goldblatt?"

"So far," I said.

"We're just going to hook you up to a drip. You tell us if you're uncomfortable."

The nurse put the IV in my left arm and said, in a sweet voice, "Now I want you to count down from one hundred to ninety. Can you do that?"

"I think so."

"All right, start."

"One hundred, ninety-nine . . ."

"You're done," Doctor P said.

"What?"

"You're done. You can roll over."

I rolled over. "Done with what?"

"Your colonoscopy."

"Yeah. Okay. What?"

"It's over," he said, smiling.

"What's over?"

"The procedure. It's over."

"Oh. What?"

"Everything looks good," he said. "We'll wait for the test results, but I don't see any problems."

Linda was waiting for me in the front office. She immediately pointed out that I'd buttoned my shirt wrong, and that only half of it was tucked in. Then she began to laugh. "You're *so* buzzed!"

"I'm not buzzed," I mumbled. "I'm fine."

"C'mon, let's get out of here and operate some heavy machinery."

She took me home in a cab, walked me up to my apartment, tucked me into my bed, and I slept for roughly the rest of January.

Doctor P turned out to be right. My colon got a clean bill of health. Unfortunately, that left the rest of me unaccounted for and back at square one with my symptoms. As I discussed these with Doctor P during our follow-up visit, he smiled sympathetically. He didn't seem put off by the discussion in the least, and I was grateful for his professionalism, though I'm sure he was hot-showering on the inside. He told me he wanted to do a full battery of tests that afternoon.

Blood test.

I nodded.

Urine test.

I nodded.

Stool sample.

"You know, my symptoms aren't really *that* bad . . ."

"Are you willing to live like this the rest of your life?"

"How long is that anyway? Twenty-five years, tops . . ."

"All right," he said. "But let me just give you the kit."

I took the kit home and prayed, for the next several days, that the blood or urine tests would provide a clear-cut answer. The call came. Both tests had turned up negative. I closed my eyes. I knew what was coming. Doctor P's voice lowered over the phone. "So I guess it's your move."

There are current as well as archaic expressions that describe how I spent the week that followed. Gearing myself up. Girding my loins. Screwing my courage to the sticking place. Putting on my big-girl panties. Taking the bull by the horns. Stepping up to the plate.

The plate, by the way, is not included in the "kit"—which consists of a pair of plastic vials the size of rifle shells, a pair of plastic spoons the size of Pinkberry tasters, and a pair of plastic gloves the size of, well, plastic gloves. But a paper plate—a stiff, substantial one, not a cheap pizza parlor job—is necessary, because the sample cannot hit the water.

Which means it has to be intercepted.

Having come this far, I don't think I'll describe the contortions and indignities I went through to acquire the sample. Suffice it to say, I stepped up to the plate. Again, however, tests revealed nothing.

Doctor P said, "Looks like we're down to trial and error."

The first week, we tried a diet of high fiber.

My symptoms persisted.

The second week, we tried low fiber.

My symptoms persisted.

The third week, we tried high carbs.

My symptoms persisted.

The fourth week, we tried low carbs.

My symptoms persisted.

The fifth week, we tried gluten-free.

I was cured.

It was an affirmation of Aristotelian logic, of cause and effect. Three days into a gluten-free diet, and my digestive track was back in perfect working order, humming along like workshop full of enzyme-enriched elves.

So now I knew: I had a gluten sensitivity.

My first reaction was relief, tinged with shame. Gluten sensitivity? I mean, it just seemed so . . . dainty. Here I was, thinking I had something dire, something acidic slowly and steadily making mincemeat of my insides, like an ulcer or maybe even a tapeworm, and instead it turned out I'd been laid low for months by *wheat*. How could that be? I mean, I was always the guy who ate the black peppers in Tang's Marvelous Beef, who ordered his Buffalo chicken sandwich extra spicy. How could *that* guy be undone by a couple of crackers? Set aside the gluten thing for a moment.. . . I'd been undone by a *sensitivity*? Not even a legit allergy, which would've shown up in the blood work, let alone celiac disease—a genuinely desperate and debilitating digestive reflex that could've brought Lou Gehrig to his knees. No, I had a whole grain *ow-wee*. I had a bread-basket *boo-boo*.

Still, now at least I knew what was wrong. Adjustments had to be made. Doctor P emailed me several web links and attached a PDF called "Living Gluten Free." Following instructions, I immediately threw out two boxes of unfrosted strawberry Pop-Tarts a loaf of Irish soda bread, and an Entenmann's pound cake . . . the first three items on my kitchen counter. (The Irish soda bread was especially heartbreaking; I'd just bought it, and Saint Patrick's Day was right around the corner.) By the time I finished reading ingredient labels and tossing groceries a half hour later, nothing was left on the kitchen counter except salt and pepper shakers, and the only things left in my refrigerator were a carton of skim milk and a jar of olives. And they were glaring at each other accusingly.

Ridding my kitchen of gluten was the easy part.

Ridding my diet of gluten was far more complicated. On a typical weekday, I ate a strawberry Pop-Tart or a bowl of Froot Loops for breakfast, a slice of pizza or a bagel and cream cheese for lunch, and a Subway sandwich or Chinese noodle takeout for dinner. Toss in an occasional turkey burger to break the monotony, and that pretty much covered my Monday through Friday. The weekends? Pasta and more pasta. The whole of it, from tart to tortellini, was now *verboten*. What to substitute? I don't eat eggs. I don't eat fish. I *do* eat certain kinds of sushi—cucumber rolls, avocado rolls, and California rolls. But it turns out that soy sauce, into which the sushi is dipped (or else, I ask you, what's the point?) isn't safe because farmers who grow soybeans often rotate their crops with—*wait for it*—wheat.

I became acquainted with a brave new world of gluten-free foodstuffs. It's a full-blown industry, led by a company called Glutino, whose mission statement is downright evangelical:

> To embrace a gluten free life is to embrace a bountiful life. A life filled with possibility and opportunity. A life unhampered by "can't" and "don't" and "won't." A life where our bodies and hearts and minds are balanced and in tune. . . . And living is what it's all about. Living everyday with joy and freedom and confidence. On our own terms. In our own way. . . . But there can be side effects to living gluten free. Chronic euphoria is

pretty common. You might experience regular bouts of giddiness along with a skin condition we like to refer to as the gluten free glow. If symptoms persist, try not to gloat.

Since my life has been a continuous procession of "can't," "don't," and "won't," I was anxious to explore the bold, sentence-fragmented promise of the Glutino brand. The first product I tried was their Seeded Bread. It had the outward appearance of traditional bread, with the taste and consistency of dried caulk. When I spread peanut butter on it, it tore. When I put roasted chicken on it, it fractured. When I toasted it, it hissed and began to spark.

Glutino toaster pastries—the GF answer to Pop-Tarts—are kind of like paperback books stuffed with molten jam. Their pretzels are delicately salted splinters of balsa wood; their chips are shards of tree bark.

To be fair, Glutino does much better in the cookie field. Their chocolate-covered wafer sticks are addictive, and their vanilla Oreo variant could make the angels weep (while clogging their celestial arteries). Glutino frozen dinners, measured against other frozen dinners, are nothing to write home about. But if you don't mind frozen dinners—which, I realize, eliminates a large swath of the public—chances are you're not going to miss the gluten.

Some foods, of course, are gluten-free in their natural form. Fruits and vegetables, for example. (Hate 'em.) Beef and poultry. (Was weaning myself from red meat when The Change happened. Now herds cower at my name.) Candies, insofar as they have a natural form, are hit-and-miss on the gluten front. Three Musketeers can be enjoyed to the hilt, but Milky Way is a no-fly zone. The promise of a slightly chilled Peppermint Pattie has gotten me through many a wilted lettuce wrap. The fact that our universe contains the necessary ingredients for both milk chocolate and peanut butter has always struck me as evidence of intelligent design; the fact that Reese's Peanut Butter Cups are certified GF now strikes me as evidence of a loving God.

On the whole, however, the GF lifestyle is not the heaviest cross to bear. I can, as the saying goes, live with it. What I *do* resent is the palpable suspicion among friends and acquaintances that I *elected* to go gluten-free. By coincidence, my divorce from wheat occurred at the exact moment that the GF diet achieved fad status; it's the intolerance of the new millennium—unless you count the media's disdain for Mormonism—which makes this the first time I've ever ridden a wave of conspicuous non-consumption.

Even more unsettling is the thought that, from a strictly Darwinian standpoint, I may not be fit to survive. The grain that sustained the Fertile Crescent, that signaled the dawn of civilization, has become my downfall. Shouldn't the likes of me therefore have perished long ago—perhaps somewhere around Olduvai Gorge, standing off to the side with Lactose-Intolerant Woman, our pee pees and hoo hoos hopelessly mismatched, as the parade of wonder-enriched homos passed us by?

I mean, isn't that what natural selection is all about?

SOFTBALL SHTICK

One of the odder phenomena of middle age, or rather of *my* middle age, is that certain Yiddish expressions have started to come back to me. Or rather *come* to me—since only about six words of Yiddish were ever spoken in the Goldblatt household, and only for emphasis rather than for meaning, and since the last time I set foot in a synagogue, except to meet a social obligation, was on the morning of my bar mitzvah. It's quite a mystical thing to have artifacts of another language, a dying language, zoom into your head out of the collective unconscious of your race, or perhaps just out of the ether.

For example, I was playing softball in Flushing Meadow Park several summers ago, standing in the sunny isolation of center field, when a hard ground ball took two hops across the infield, struck a pebble and bounced straight up into our third baseman's groin. I winced as he fell to the ground, and, an instant later, thought: "*Oy*, right in *de shvantz*!" Then, after five minutes, when at last his girlfriend came running back to the ball field with a plastic bag full of ice, from deep within the *kishkes* of my brain, what occurred to me was: "*'Svet gornisht helfen.*" I didn't even know what the expression meant until I tracked it down, that night, on the Internet. It seems to be a cross between "too little too late" and "it's not going to help one bit." How it came to me, or why it came to me, I've not a clue. But if it turns out that circumcision is more than a physical token, more than *a little bit off the top*, as we used to say in the 'hood, if indeed I am haunted by the ghosts of *shtetls* past, well, then, so be it.

But to return to our stricken third baseman, whom I'll call Sheldon, since that is in fact his name, the aforementioned bad hop caught him in the final inning of a tied game against our archrivals, the Zoo. Ah, the cursèd Zoo! They were a nasty but well-named lot, culled from the lifetime subscription list for *Easyriders* magazine and the toxic end of Hulk Hogan's gene pool. They were the Hatfields to our McCoys, the Montagues to our Capulets, the Philistines to our Israelites. Their game plan was elemental; their lumbering, pot-bellied and occasionally inebriated batters belched and farted their way into the batter's box, then swung from their heels with the pent-up rage that lurks beneath every Serenity prayer. By contrast, our team was built on speed, defense, and an occasional Fresca; we ran down their long drives deep in the outfield, and we took extra bases whenever their fielders didn't hustle after the ball. The Zoo hated us for our first-to-third dashes, for our savvy situational hitting, for our copies of the *New York Times* Book Review tucked into our equipment bags, for our wives' and girlfriends' shaved legs and full sets of teeth, for our discernable necks and prehensile thumbs.

All of that was forgotten, however, as Sheldon went down. Both teams, within moments, gathered around third-base. Sympathetic glances were exchanged. Hands were placed on rivals' shoulders. As Sheldon lay writhing in the dirt, the Zoo catcher knelt down beside him and whispered tenderly, barely audibly, "You'll be all right, guy. Just stay still." Would a torn tendon have elicited such compassion from a ham-fisted brute whose nickname, sewn into the back of his jersey, was Hondo? Not likely. Would a separated shoulder have so stirred the australopithecine heart that beat beneath his team's block-lettered insignia? Again, no. The sight of a splintered, jagged femur jutting through the flesh of Sheldon's thigh . . . Hondo would've told him to rub dirt on it, then turned to the umpire and called, "Yo, Blue, can the dude play or not?"

But a shot to the groin is different . . . perhaps because all ballplayers have been there. It's part of the game, as much as cursing and spitting and patting your teammates on the butt. The ball, having been struck over and over by the bat, suddenly decides to take revenge on the bat's little brother. Even the aesthetics are painful to contemplate. The momentum-rich heft of the ball. The come-and-get-me posture of the penile shaft. The winking eye. The ball-field euphemism for a shot to the groin is taking one in the family jewels. I rather like that expression, the pomp and circumstance of it, the sudden breach of protocol, the crest and scepter rattling with synecdoche.

I've taken one in the family jewels at least a half dozen times over the years. It's a mystical experience that can be conceived in distinct stages. First comes the *oomph*, the shock, the sickening warmth, the waves of nausea that roll upward through your chest and break into foam at the back of your throat. Then you think: *I'm going to die*. Then you think: *I'm going to live*. Then you think: *Maybe that's not such a good thing*. But in the end, you're all right. The loyal soldier has fallen; the war goes on. Your teammates help you back to the bench. You sit there, slumped forward, your head parallel to your knees, and you listen to their good-natured ribbing, "Hey, your kids would've been ugly anyway."

Shots to the groin are flukes, however. The more common injuries are scrapes and bruises—and these are the bane of the middle-aged softball player. Last fall, for example, as the season was winding down, on a morning so cold that I was wearing every spare undergarment I owned, including the tallit I got for my bar mitzvah, and with a dog-neutering wind whipping across the field, I singled the potential tying run to third in the last inning. There was one out. Our chances looked good, but the next batter was Gasper, the slowest runner on the team. So I knew what Michael, the first-base coach, was about to tell me.

"Don't even say it," I said to him. "I'm not going to slide."

"You have to slide if he hits a ground ball—"

"I'm *not* going to slide."

"You have to break up the double play on a ground ball."

"Then he better not hit a ground ball, because I'm not sliding."

There was an awkward pause.

"Look," I muttered, "he probably won't hit a ground ball."

"But if he does," Michael said, "you *are* going to slide, right?"

"No, I'm not going to—"

I couldn't finish the sentence because the pitcher had let go of the ball, and Gasper had hit a hard grounder right at the second baseman. As I sprinted toward the bag, I was thinking, *No way. It's not worth it. Nothing on this earth can make me slide. I don't get paid to play this game. I'm not going to slide. . . .* Then I slid. What I pictured was one of those quick sit-down scoots, the kind where you pop up at the base, where you raise just enough dust to distract the infielders—the kind of slide Vince Coleman used to specialize in when he wasn't getting eaten by tarps or injuring toddlers with fireworks. The problem, however, was that I never committed to the slide; I didn't slide so much as crumble in stages. As the shortstop hopped over me to complete his throw to first, I could feel swatches of skin peeling away from my right hip, my right elbow, and my right palm. I heard the umpire call Gasper out, then took a quick inventory of internal organs. Nothing seemed ruptured. But there was a lot of sloshing around. The shortstop, who was young enough to be my biological son, except my biological son wouldn't have been playing shortstop, thrust out his hand to help me up. The look on his face read, "Yikes, that must hurt."

As he hauled me to my feet, I caught myself thinking: *Oy, de* pain!

Notwithstanding the fact that I've played organized softball for the last three decades, that I've sustained two broken collarbones, six fractured fingers, thirty-seven pulled hamstrings, and one AstroTurf burn on my left calf that took nine months to heal, that I've sacrificed promising romances and glorious vacations abroad on the altar of the Goddess Clincher, truth be told, I've never been more than a run-of-the-mill player. That judgment, of course, must be understood in context. Put me in a weekend pickup game—you know, just folks out to have fun at the company picnic—and I'll shine like a new penny. But the trained eye will notice defects. The coordination between my hands and my eyes is erratic and fraught with mutually exclusive agendas. My throwing arm has been reported to Colonel Sanders and compared unfavorably to a lo mein noodle, and my batting swing would make a rusty gate creak with shame. Indeed, I'd have long ago been relegated to the role of benchwarmer, or else chucked outright, save for the fact that I'm an unnaturally fast runner and thus have a continued canine value in the outfield. As my longtime teammate Sal once uncharitably observed, the only sport in which I could have gone pro was fetch.

Still, the end is nigh. To be nothing but fast is to be helpless as your speed goes into decline. There is no skill I can master at this stage of my softball life to compensate, no cagey veteran adjustments I can make. Strive though I might to take each season one game at a time, to beat back the idea of retirement by shutting my eyes and repeating to myself "la-la-la-la-la-la," cost-benefit analyses have begun to worm their way into my thoughts. Even now, the ratio of time I spend preparing to play a game—stretching my hamstring and calf muscles, gulping down ibuprofens, wrapping my thighs to gangrene-defying pressures and smearing palmfuls of Bengay on whichever joints I can still reach—compared with the time I spend actually playing nears one to one. Worse still is the game's aftermath. First comes the unraveling—a kind of reverse mummification that ends with streamers of beige and white ace bandages fluttering in the wind at my side. Next is the de-cleating. This is bad because it involves bending forward and making universal old-man noises: *Urrrgh. Unnngh. Nummnh.* Then comes the lingering blank stare as the inner adult silently engages the inner child. Their debate runs along predictable lines: "It's not worth it anymore." "Oh, come on, it's still fun!" "No one's paying you to do this." "But it's good exercise! It keeps you in shape!" "Are you an idiot? Look at yourself!" "Please, please, please, just five more minutes! I'll be good the rest of the week!"

Once I get home, further torments await. Underneath my uniform, I wear a skin-tight thermal shirt—which gets soaked with sweat. Pulling it off over my head entails a contortion act that would have set Houdini's teeth on edge and often winds up with the thermal shirt inside out but still tight around my neck, and with me careening blindly around the apartment, knocking over floor lamps and tray tables. Then comes the ritual application of ice packs to shoulders and knees, followed a half hour later by a hot bath in which the ongoing challenge is to remain conscious; I cannot count the times I've awakened in the tub just as my chin and nose slid below the waterline, coughing up mouthfuls of Epsom salt.

The reader might be forgiven at this point for rolling his eyes at the *kvetching* of a middle-aged man who hit the circumstantial jackpot of being born in America, in decent health, and with enough wits about him to cobble together a life that has allowed him to play organized softball for three decades. So what if my moment in the sun is passing?

Except what I'm *kvetching* about, if the reader hasn't figured it out yet, isn't the transience of softball but the transience of existence. The dwindling of my playing days is a foreshadowing of the dwindling of my days, the petering out of the life force underneath the uniform, underneath the sun-creased skin, underneath the sinew and cartilage that fail with greater and greater frequency.

I am in ebb mode.

Here is a confession: I used to keep a guitar pick in my pocket. I told friends it was a good-luck charm, a sentimental token, but in truth I kept it around just in case an Elvis Presley movie broke out, and I had to win back Ann-Margaret's heart with a song. That was how I thought of myself. Center stage. Spotlighted. Mic'd up. The audience hanging on my every sneer and glance. But that image is no longer sustainable. Pausing in front of a mirror, I'm confronted by the truth that if an Elvis Presley movie *did* break out, I'd be the old guy, the William Demarest character, who leans out the window and tells the kids to knock off the racket.

I do not think they will sing to me.

How did it happen? One minute ago, or so it seemed, I was strutting and fretting, a poor player perhaps but a player nevertheless, and now, a minute later, I'm an attendant lord, *noodging* and *kibitzing*, swelling a progress in the Yiddish Theater. Now I stand at a podium in front of a college classroom and give lectures on the Old Testament, and bored coeds crane their necks at the sunlight streaming in through the windows. Literally, they are leaning into it. Spring is right up in their faces. It's quickening their blood. The temperature outside is seventy degrees, without a hint of humidity. There's a breeze they can hear but not feel. *Why oh why*, they are thinking, *won't this geezer shut up about the Book of Job*?

Then, too, there's the whole mortality thing. Bad enough that I never played center field for the New York Yankees, the first of my many career options—astronaut, rock star, secret agent, Olympic sprinter—to fizzle out. Now the sports heroes of my childhood, the baseball and football and basketball players whose posters once hung on my bedroom wall, are dying of natural causes. Even among my peers, my lifelong friends, Death has begun to *nosh*. He takes a breast, part of a lung, a hunk of kidney. So far, I've eluded his attention. But how much longer can that last?

Because the lineup is moving. Inexorably, the lineup is moving. From the shade of the dugout, I watched my father step to the plate against the Eternal Windmiller; I watched him take his hacks and go down swinging. Three quick risers, and he was done. Then I watched my mother's turn; she worked the count full, fouled off pitch after pitch, until in the end she looked at a called third strike on a nasty change-up. I don't remember moving to the on-deck circle while she was batting, but I must have, because now the umpire is pointing his finger straight at me, motioning me into the box. And I'm glancing around, listening to catcalls from the sparse crowd, helplessly and hopelessly *farblondzhet*.

I know I can't hit this guy.

ACKNOWLEDGMENTS

I find myself once again in the debt of Adam Bellow, whose belief in this book—notwithstanding my lack of a reality TV show and the fact that I come up 99,937 short of 100,000 Twitter followers—has rescued it from obscurity. Through Adam, I have become indebted, as well, to the Liberty Island crew: David Bernstein, David Swindle, and Elena Vega.

My agent, Scott Gould, of RLR Associates, who first alerted me to the difficulty of finding a home for a book of funny narrative essays without aforesaid TV show or Twitter celebrity, stuck with this project—as he has several of my quirkier books. *Semper fab.*

Many of these stories began as random conversations and extended whines to which Linda Helble was subjected . . . in their unpolished forms. The fact that I am not riddled with stab wounds is a testament to her patience and sympathy.

CPSIA information can be obtained
at www.ICGtesting.com
Printed in the USA
BVOW03s2154160217
476450BV00001B/12/P

9 781504 042246